A GUIDE TO BETTER

MOVEMENT

THE **SCIENCE** AND **PRACTICE** OF **MOVING**
WITH *MORE* SKILL AND *LESS* PAIN

TODD HARGROVE, CR, CFP

A Guide to Better Movement
Copyright © 2014 by Todd R. Hargrove

For information about this title or to order other books and/or electronic media, contact the publisher:

Better Movement
2113 NE 65th Street, Seattle, WA 98115
bettermovement.org

ISBN: 978-0-9915423-0-7

Printed in the United States of America

Cover and Interior design by: 1106 Design

Thanks to photographer Paul Joseph Brown and model Rose Wetzel-Sinnett

Disclaimer:
All forms of exercise carry some risk. Readers are advised to take full responsibility for their safety and their limits. The advice in this book is in no way intended to be a substitute for any advice provided by your doctor or other medical professional. The information in this book is true and correct to the best of the author's knowledge. However, science is always advancing, and therefore the information may become outdated or proven incorrect. The author and publisher disclaim all liability for damages caused by doing the lessons or applying the recommendations in this book.

ACKNOWLEDGMENTS

THERE ARE MANY PEOPLE I would like to thank for making this book possible.

Thanks to my teachers, colleagues, and clients for providing information, good ideas, criticism, and encouragement. In particular:

Paul Ingraham, Tony Ingram, Jason Silvernail, Diane Jacobs, Barrett Dorko, Greg Lehman, Michael Reoch, Alice Sanvito, Carol Lynn Chevrier, Will Stewart, Matthew Danziger, Chris Johnson, Michael Li, Nick Tuminello, Bret Contreras, Eric Cressey, Charlie Weingroff, Patrick Ward, Joel Jamieson, Phillip Snell, Gray Cook, Mike Boyle, Shirley Sahrmann, Craig Liebenson, Pavel Kolar, Stu McGill, Paul Hodges, Lorimer Moseley, David Butler, Tom Myers, Eric Cobb, Moshe Feldenkrais, Jeff Haller, Richard Corbeil, Frank Wildman, Dwight Pargee, Mabel Todd, Geoffrey Bove, Chris Highcock, Rafe Kelly, Seth Will, Stephan Guyenet, Brad Jones, Steven Pinker, Richard Dawkins, Nikolai Bernstein, Mel Siff. And many others!

And thanks to my family and friends for their love and support, especially Jemila, Juniper and Abezash.

TABLE OF CONTENTS

PREFACE

I GREW UP PLAYING SPORTS. Organized sports, disorganized sports, team sports and individual sports. I played baseball and basketball through middle school, soccer through high school, and tennis through college. Even though upstate New York is not exactly a hotbed for college tennis, I was proud to play at the top spot for a few years.

I was always very interested in what made the good players good. Was it size, speed, strength, skill, conditioning? Was it practice or innate skill?

I became far more interested in these subjects when I started competing at pool in college. I'm not sure why. Perhaps it's because in pool, there are no obvious physical barriers to playing just as well as the pros. You don't need to be big, strong, or fast. You just need to hit the ball in the right place at the right speed.

Whatever the case, I became a little obsessed about playing professional-level pool. I bought every book I could find, and I watched videotapes of the pros for hours to analyze their technique. My friends thought this was pretty weird. Hard to blame them!

During this process, I discovered I have an unusual interest in watching movement, analyzing it, and figuring out how to emulate it. As a result, I became a pretty good pool player. (But not a pro!)

I soon learned I could become similarly interested in other physical activities. In my twenties I took up squash, and eventually won the A flight of the Seattle Open three times.

During the same time I was learning about movement, I was also, unfortunately, learning about chronic pain. In my twenties I spent a lot of time working at a computer as a law student and attorney, and this probably contributed to chronic pain in my neck, shoulders, and low back. My knees and feet hurt too. I felt like I was getting old in the prime of my life.

When I was in pain, I couldn't focus on my work. Or play sports competitively. Or enjoy sitting at a movie, or going on a long car ride. My sleep suffered and I just *never* felt truly comfortable or at home in my body.

I began reading large volumes of mostly conflicting information about what causes pain and how to treat it. I went to doctors, physical therapists, classes in yoga and Pilates. I read extensively about corrective exercise, functional training, posture, stretching, medical and alternative approaches to pain treatment. I soon realized that I found chronic pain to be a fascinating topic, even aside from its practical application to my life. And that I could become just as absorbed in the study of pain as I was in the study of performance. I also noticed many interesting connections between these seemingly different topics.

As a result, I made very steady progress over a few years until I eliminated my chronic pain. That was more than twelve years ago. I'm now forty-six, continue to compete at sports, and feel terrific in my body. I get hurt from time to time, but I know how to get better. All in all, I feel better now than I did in my twenties, which makes me very optimistic about the potential for change we all have. I know it's not all about getting old.

In 2005, I decided to quit being an attorney and find a career that was more aligned with my interests. I became a Rolfer and Feldenkrais practitioner and have been working in Seattle with clients since then.

In 2008, I started writing a blog to help family, friends, and clients better understand what I learned about pain and movement through my practice and research. Part of my intention was to correct common misconceptions that I see in people who have pain.

If someone in pain goes to a physical therapist, family doctor, surgeon, chiropractor, acupuncturist, personal trainer, or massage therapist, he or she might receive seven different explanations for their pain, and seven completely different treatments. And there is a very good chance many of these explanations or treatments will not be supported by any good science at all. Or even worse, in direct conflict with science! I saw people getting confused, distressed, and wasting time and resources.

There is a common theme in this confusion. Many therapists overemphasize the extent to which some alleged defect in the body is responsible for pain. For example, pain might be blamed on bad posture, imbalanced chi, a misaligned spine, a weak core, short hip flexors, muscle knots, or a bulging disc. At the same time, the role of the nervous system and the brain is neglected or misunderstood.

This is ironic because it is quite often the nervous system, and not some assumed pathology in the body, that actually changes for the better during a successful treatment. In fact, it is very likely that when someone feels better — after a chiropractic adjustment, a yoga session, foam rolling, acupuncture, massage, or corrective exercise — very similar mechanisms are at play. And this is true even though the practitioners might imagine they are aiming at completely different targets. Recent advances in pain science and neuroscience provide significant insight into these mechanisms and how they can be most effectively accessed.

So the theme of my blog (and this book) is:

* In order to maximize the benefit of any practice intended to help us move better and feel better, we need to understand the actual mechanisms at play.

* The nervous system has far more control over perceptions and movements of the body than most people imagine.

* The fastest and easiest way to start moving better and feeling better is to make changes in the nervous system.

After writing on these subjects for a year or two, I was amazed to see my blog was getting attention and positive reviews from many nationally known physical therapists and athletic trainers. Several teachers of physical therapy, yoga, or martial arts wrote to me and told me they were referring their students to my articles. I found my posts linked by some of my favorite bloggers. My readership grew until I was in regular contact with a large network of very educated and intelligent people. As a result, my knowledge and commitment to providing accurate and accessible information increased exponentially.

By 2012, I decided to write this book to organize and build on the various ideas I had discussed on the blog. I hope you find the information in this book to be as fascinating and useful as I did.

INTRODUCTION

IF YOU ARE READING THIS BOOK, you are probably someone who wants to learn to move better and feel better. Maybe you are an athlete, a chronic pain sufferer, or someone who enjoys mind-body practices for personal development or self-discovery. Maybe you are a professional devoted to helping others with their movement: a physical therapist, massage therapist, chiropractor, personal trainer, or instructor in yoga, Pilates, or martial arts.

If so, this book is for you. It explains the fascinating science related to moving with skill and comfort, and it provides practical strategies to accomplish these goals. The focus of this book is on the nervous system — how it controls the way we move and feel. One major theme is that it has far more influence on strength, speed, flexibility, endurance, pain, and coordination than you might imagine.

I tried to write this book with enough scientific detail to please movement professionals, while at the same time remaining accessible to readers with no pre-existing knowledge of the subject matter. With that in mind, I have several goals.

First, to provide a science based yet common sense framework for understanding motor control and its relationship to performance, pain, and personal well-being. The hopeful result is a simple lens through which to understand a large amount of complex and seemingly contradictory information from many different fields, all of which use their own vocabulary and concepts. After reading this book, you will be better able to synthesize ideas from

1

separate fields, simplify ideas that are complex, clarify ideas that are fuzzy, and discard ideas that are nonsense.

The second goal of this book is to articulate some general principles that can be used to improve *any* program that uses movement to reduce pain or increase physical performance. Whether you do yoga, Pilates, physical therapy, or corrective exercise, this book can help you understand exactly why what you are doing works, and how to make things work better.

The third goal of this book is to provide some movement lessons that apply the science and principles discussed in the preceding sections. The last chapter includes twenty-five movement lessons that are based on the Feldenkrais Method, each of which focuses on improving a fundamental function such as reaching, locomotion, or coordinating the legs with the trunk. If you haven't been previously exposed to Feldenkrais, you will find these lessons unique, interesting, fun, challenging and beneficial. And an ideal way to explore movement on your own, without a coach or teacher.

Why Better Movement?

Given that you are reading this book, I assume you are already convinced that improving the quality of your movement is a worthwhile goal. In the event that you need more convincing, here are three primary reasons that working to improve the efficiency, coordination and comfort of your movement may be beneficial.

1. Performance and injury prevention

The best athletes, the best dancers, the best martial artists and yogis are not just those who are the strongest, fastest or most flexible. (Although all those things help!) The best are those with the highest *quality* of movement, the best coordination, the best organization of the body. What sets them apart — people like Tiger Woods, Roger Federer, Leo Messi, and Mia Hamm — is not their size, strength and speed, but their movement intelligence.

Movement quality is also what helps elite performers stay free of injury. If you train hard enough to get good at anything, you will put your body under a tremendous amount of mechanical stress. Efficient movement helps one avoid injury by minimizing and distributing the mechanical stress of movement.

2. Comfort in activities of daily living

The way you move affects how you feel as you go through the activities of everyday life. Even a sedentary life is completely filled with physical activity — sitting, standing, walking, breathing, reaching, bending, etc. Sitting at a computer is a demanding task that causes many injuries. We are all athletes whether we know it or not.

Just as in sport, the movements of everyday life can be performed with more or less coordination and efficiency. Habitual use of excess tension or mechanical stress in these activities is unlikely to cause any discomfort over the course of a minute or two, but accumulated over the course of days, weeks and years, the effects may become significant. Learning better movement may help avoid or reduce chronic pain and stress.

Of course the body is very adaptable and we do not need each of our movements to be biomechanically perfect in order to avoid pain and have good function. And indeed many people with seemingly inefficient movement patterns have no pain and vice versa. However, movement is one of many sources of stress in life, and we would rather have less stress than more. Sometimes it makes a critical difference.

3. Personal development

Moving better is not just about moving better. The parts of your brain that control movement are linked to the parts that control thoughts, emotions and sensory perceptions. If you want to change your emotional or mental state, and indeed your self-image, changing the way you perceive and move your body is one way to go about it. Movement is a concrete handle that can be used to grasp more abstract and intangible qualities of the brain.

This is why many traditional forms of movement therapy such as yoga, Pilates, martial arts, tai chi, and the Feldenkrais Method are intended to bring health to the mind as much to the body.

A Brain-Based Perspective

This book has a "brain-based" perspective. That means the focus is on how the central nervous system affects how we move and feel, and what we can do to change its function in that regard.

This does not imply the structure of the body is unimportant, or good movement is "all in your head." Far from it! The structure and health of the musculoskeletal system is essential for quality movement, just as a mechanically sound car is required for safe driving.

But there are many books on how to improve the structure of the body through various forms of diet, exercise and stress reduction. By contrast, there are far fewer books addressing how we can optimize the function of the nervous system, which controls the body. And many people in the field of optimizing movement do not fully appreciate the extent to which the nervous system plays a role in issues of strength, speed, flexibility, endurance, coordination and pain. This book is an attempt to provide some much needed balance in the way therapists and trainers look at movement.

Distinguishing hardware and software

If you want to fix a computer that has crashed, you need to know if the problem is in the hardware or the software. If you want to know why a car crashed, you might ask whether the fault lies with the car or the driver. Did the car run off the road because the tires failed, or because the driver was not careful enough? If a guitar doesn't sound right, is it because the instrument is out of tune, or because the player is not hitting the right notes?

We can ask similar questions when looking at human movement. If your hip flexors feel tight while running, is that because they are too short, or just unable to relax? Is it because your glutes are atrophied in their size, or just inhibited in their function? And if you have hip pain while running, is that because of damage in the hip, or a nervous system that has become overly sensitized to normal movement? Is the problem structure or function, muscle or nervous system, car or driver, hardware or software?

Admittedly, we cannot always answer this question, or even draw a bright line between structure and function. The distinction is sometimes more of an abstract concept than an objective anatomical reality. Nevertheless, these concepts can be a useful thinking tool for understanding why movement is problematic, and what needs to be targeted to make an improvement.

As stated above, this book will focus on interventions that affect function not structure, the software not the hardware, the driver not the car, the player not the instrument. There are several very good reasons to make sure we are maximizing the function of the nervous system as we try to improve movement. Here are three.

The nervous system is highly adaptable

The central nervous system is in many ways more plastic and adaptable than the structure of the body. Some structural changes are effectively impossible to make. Bones only change their shape and density over the course of many years, and we are therefore pretty much stuck with the skeletons that we have grown into by the time we are adults.

The length of our soft tissues is also not easy to change. Although we might imagine we are lengthening muscle by stretching, it is more likely that increased range of motion is caused by changes in the nervous system's *tolerance* to stretch, rather than actual length changes in muscles.[1]

Similarly, therapies intended to lengthen or alter fascia probably do not work by changing its structure, but instead through effects on the nervous system. Research shows the forces required to deform mature connective tissue are probably impossible to create with hands, elbows or foam rollers.[2] Although connective tissue does respond to mechanical stress, change is a long slow process similar to building bones.

In contrast to the structure of the body, functional changes have almost unlimited potential. If you want to become a better basketball player, there is not much you can do to change your height, but there is vast potential to learn basketball skills with the right kind of practice. And the emerging science of neuroplasticity is proving the brain is capable of reorganization throughout its lifetime.

The nervous system can change very quickly

The structure of the body changes very slowly in response to accumulated stress. Over the course of years, bones that are repeatedly struck in the same place will eventually get harder and denser. Ligaments and tendons that are repeatedly stressed to a certain level will grow stronger and thicker over the course of months. When muscles are tested enough they will grow larger, and this will take at least a few weeks. All these adaptations improve function and reduce damage from mechanical stress.

While these changes are interesting and very important, they are almost idiotically slow and simple in comparison to the complex adaptability of the nervous system. When the nervous system detects excess mechanical stress in the body, it takes a wide variety of corrective actions *instantly*. It will immediately reorganize movement patterns to shift stress away from endangered areas. It can create pain to protect those areas further. It can change perception to provide more precise control of movement. And over the course of only a few minutes, it can learn new ways to move that are safer and more efficient.

Thus, the central nervous system is incredibly sensitive and responsive to information in the environment. It can change in an instant, and the brain can learn new skills rapidly. If you are feeling and moving better after a session of yoga, massage, or corrective exercise, it is highly likely the relevant changes have occurred more in the nervous system than the structure of the body.

Nervous system changes can be permanent

Functional adaptations of the central nervous system have another potential advantage over physical adaptations like gains in muscle size. When developed to a certain level, learning by the central nervous system is effectively permanent. Although we can easily lose the muscles or fitness gained through weight training during time off from the gym, we never forget how to ride a bike. Similarly, the lessons about body awareness and coordination that can be learned through the practice of yoga, martial arts, the Feldenkrais method, or other mindfulness-based movement therapies can potentially benefit the user for a long period of time, provided they are learned to sufficient degree.

Roadmap

With this background in mind, let's take a quick look at the organization of this book, which has three parts. Part I covers the science of movement, Part II focuses on pain and other protective mechanisms, and Part III is about putting these ideas into practice. Following is a chapter by chapter breakdown.

Part I: The Science of Moving Better

Chapter 1 defines the essential qualities of movements that are biomechanically most healthy, efficient, functional or otherwise desirable.

Chapter 2 discusses how the nervous system perceives and controls movement, and how we can learn to control it better.

Chapter 3 is about "maps" in the brain — patterns of neural activity that represent the body and help govern movement and perception. We will look at how they change and why it matters.

Chapter 4 views movement from a developmental perspective, looking at the fundamental building blocks for movement that we learned as toddlers, and the value of developmental positions for recovering and maintaining fundamental movement patterns as adults.

Part II: The Science of Feeling Better

Chapter 5 discusses the role of the brain in creating pain, why pain does not equal tissue damage, and the way pain is affected by our thoughts and emotions.

Chapter 6 discusses protective mechanisms or "central governors" that may limit our physical performance. Stiffness, weakness, fatigue and altered coordination are all ways the nervous system protects us from movements perceived to be threatening.

Chapter 7 provides a scientific framework for understanding how various mind-body disciplines promote self-improvement and emotional control.

Part III: The Practice of Moving Better and Feeling Better

Chapter 8 uses the background established in previous chapters to set forth some brain-based strategies to move better and feel better. These can be used in a wide variety of contexts.

Chapter 9 concludes with twenty-five movement lessons that illustrate one potential application of the strategies discussed in the previous chapter.

Let's get started!

PART I

THE SCIENCE OF MOVING BETTER

CHAPTER 1

DEFINING BETTER MOVEMENT

"A movement is correct when it perfectly fits a motor problem just as a key easily opens a lock."
— Nikolai Bernstein

BEFORE WE TRY TO improve movement, we should develop some ideas about what good movement looks like. What are the essential qualities of movements that are biomechanically most healthy and functional?

This chapter will not involve detailed discussions of anatomy or assessments that are very *specific* to a *particular* movement or joint.[3] Instead, we will focus on *general* principles of good biomechanics that apply to almost every movement we make, and every person who moves. For example, to increase performance and reduce injury, it is generally true that the mechanical stress of movement should be shared by many joints, as opposed to highly concentrated in one joint. This principle remains true whether we are talking about the foot or the shoulder, running or walking, breathing or jumping, an elite athlete or an old man.

With that in mind, this chapter will try to identify the *essential* qualities of all healthy and functional movements. In the process, it will clarify some confusion that exists in regard to many concepts that are commonly used to describe movement qualities, like stability, mobility, flexibility, balance, posture, or alignment. Is flexibility important? How is it different from mobility? Does posture and core stability matter? Are there "right" and "wrong" ways to move? Read on for answers.

Before getting started, it should be acknowledged that biomechanics are not everything. As we will discuss later in the book, many people with significant chronic pain appear to have excellent movement patterns, and many people with seemingly awkward movement have no pain at all. In addition, movements and postures that are most efficient for one person might not work at all for someone else. Each person is unique and will have different optimal solutions to movement challenges.

Despite these caveats, all movements are not created equal in their relation to performance, safety and the physical stresses they create on the body. People with the highest levels of function have a lot in common in the way they move. For example, even though runners will always have some individual differences in their gaits, a group of elite runners will show less variance than novices. As Tolstoy said, "Happy families are all alike; every unhappy family is unhappy in its own way." This is true to some extent about happy movers — they share certain essential qualities in common. With that in mind, let's try to describe what these qualities might be.

Coordination

All good movement is necessarily an act of coordination, which is defined as "harmonious interaction." As applied to movements of the body, coordination means the different muscles and joints cooperate *as a team* to create a particular outcome.

Even the simplest movement requires teamwork — lifting a finger implies cooperative activity between a prime mover (it contracts to create the movement), a stabilizer (it contracts to prevent unwanted movement), and the antagonist muscle (it relaxes to allow the movement). No matter how fit or capable the individual muscles are, if they are not coordinated as a team, the movement will not occur at all.

The team analogy is useful to understand how coordination can be optimized or impaired. Many failures of coordination can be attributed to the players not cooperating, or not playing their proper positions, or a key player getting injured and sitting on the bench. Imagine turning to look over your left shoulder. Joints in the neck, shoulders, ribs and vertebrae all cooperate in turning left. What if one of the team members doesn't move at all? Other team members have to work harder to get the job done, and the efficiency of the movement is impaired.

Another useful analogy is to music — all the muscles and joints are like players in a huge orchestra. The quality of the song does not depend so much on the strength of any one note or instrument, but rather on the harmonious interaction between all the different parts of the whole. And it is important that everyone play the same tune!

Flexibility and Mobility

Good movement requires that all the joints have at least some minimum range of motion for common functions. I'm not going to define what this minimum range of motion is for each joint, which of course depends on the activity, but I will point out that the role of flexibility in good movement is generally overrated. It is also confused with a different concept called mobility, which is often more important.

Although these terms are used differently by different experts, for purposes of this book I will define flexibility as the *range of motion* at a particular joint — how far it can move from A to B. Mobility means the degree of functional control over the end range of motion. Most people need more mobility, but not more flexibility to improve their movement. In other words, they don't need more range of motion, just better performance and control at the end range they already have.

If you took an assortment of elite athletes into a lab and measured their physical qualities, you might find they had exceptional levels of strength, power, endurance or balance. But their flexibility would probably be pretty average for a healthy person. For the most part, great movement is not about how large your range of motion is, it's what you do with the range you have.

The majority of movements in sport and life take place within ranges of motion easily achievable by an average healthy person. You can prove this for yourself by looking at pictures of athletes in action. It would not be very difficult to mimic most of the joint positions displayed in the pictures. But it would be very difficult to move into these positions powerfully, smoothly, painlessly, and with the coordinated activity of other joints. These deficiencies usually have little to do with range of motion. These are issues of mobility, stability, coordination, strength, power, not flexibility.

Further, flexibility does not appear to protect against injury. For example, in hockey players, strong adductors are far more protective against groin strain than flexible adductors, which offer no benefit.[4]

But all things equal, isn't more flexibility better? Not necessarily. Flexibility in the muscles of the posterior chain correlates with slower running and poor running economy.[5] For the same reason an inflated ball bounces higher than a flat ball, tight hamstrings provide more "bounce" in running. As discussed in more detail later, excess flexibility can increase the risk of injury by destabilizing a joint.

Of course, there are some sports or physical activities where high levels of flexibility are required. Many of these involve an aesthetic element, such as dance, gymnastics, diving, or certain forms of martial arts. There is something about a large range of motion that is pleasing to the eye, and this is why dancers and gymnasts get into the splits a lot. But you won't see the splits very often in sports where there are no points awarded for style. What you will see is complete mastery over normal ranges of motion.

Stability

Stability is a major buzzword these days. People will debate which muscles are most important for creating it, whether mobility is more important or should come first, whether the lack of stability is a major source of pain, and the best ways to develop it. And the word stability is often used in the same sentence as the word "core," which is another term that tends to get people arguing. Despite these complexities, the basic meaning of the word is fairly clear. Stability simply means the ability to prevent unwanted motion.

Coordinated movement depends vitally on controlling motion, because the human body has great potential for unwanted movements. Consider the ease of controlling the movements of a door. The "joint" is the hinge, which is built in such a way to prevent the door from moving anywhere but forward or back. The structure of the joint makes the movement of the door incredibly easy to control.

The joints of the body are nothing like the hinge on a door. Each joint has many degrees of freedom, and there is significant "play" (accessory movement) in each joint. Thus, the different combinations of joint movements we can make are almost infinite. Most combinations are not useful or even safe. Therefore, most of the work of creating useful and safe movement, both energetically and in terms of the intelligence to control the movement, is in stabilizing as opposed to mobilizing.

One obviously undesirable movement is one that damages a joint. Every muscle contraction has the potential to move a hard object such as a bone into some sensitive soft tissue. For example, each time the shoulder joint absorbs a compressive force, the ball of the humerus could slide out of its socket and into some other structures. The rotator cuff muscles must create the stability to prevent this unwanted movement.

Stability is also necessary to optimize the channeling of force into a target. You may have heard the phrase, "You can't shoot a cannon out of a canoe." If the canoe is not stabilized, the force of the cannon will be wasted on moving the canoe *backward* instead of the cannonball *forward*. The same thing happens when the joint on one end of a moving bone fails to stabilize. The energy of the muscle contraction will be wasted on moving two bones instead of just one. The canoe analogy also makes clear that timing matters. Stability needs to be provided *before* the cannon fires not after.

Stability is also a prerequisite for accurate movement. Stabilizing the non-moving parts reduces the variables the brain has to deal with in predicting the consequences of muscle contractions. Imagine the difficulty of texting while riding a horse. No stability equals autocorrect disaster.

Stabilizing a joint is complex because it requires the cooperative activity of entire chains of muscle (sometimes called "slings" or "trains"). Imagine lying on your back and lifting your head from the floor to look at your feet. You can do this by contracting the muscles in the front of the neck that connect to the ribs and sternum. This contraction will pull the ribs and sternum to the head (as opposed to the head to the sternum) unless they are stabilized from below by contraction of the abdominal muscles, which connect the sternum and ribs to the pelvis. Thus, a simple movement like lifting the head requires a coordinated chain of stability.

Or imagine throwing a ball. The pectoralis major will contract to pull the arm across the body to the chest. But if the chest is not stabilized from below by the abdominal muscles, then it will move to the arm instead of acting as a fixed point to pull the arm. Preventing this type of "energy leak" is a critical aspect of coordination and efficiency in movement.

Various authors have identified numerous chains of muscle that work together during simple movements, including the posterior chain (gastrocs/soleus, hamstrings, glutes, lumbar and thoracic erectors), the lateral chain (hip abductors, quadratus lumborum, intercostals) and oblique muscle chains (interior oblique, external oblique, serratus anterior, lower trapezius, etc.).

The chains reveal that the stability required for even simple movements is highly complex and regionally interdependent. This implies that the loss of stability anywhere has the potential to affect quality of movement almost anywhere else.

Thus, complicated chains of muscle stability are required for even the simplest movements. Walk over to a doorframe and reach your left arm straight out so the palm is against the right side of the frame. Then press into the frame, as if you are trying to push it to the right. How many muscles in your body can you feel working to help you do this? You should be able to feel activity down into both feet. The quality of the stability provided by the foot and ankle can easily be felt in the hand.

A final point on stability is that is does not imply rigidity. In most cases, joints that are involved in a stability function are not completely rigid or motionless. Instead, there is usually some small amount of motion required for optimum function.

For example, although the low back vertebrae are often stabilizing themselves against unwanted movement as the extremities move, there is almost always some small amount of compensatory movement happening there to optimize function. For example, if you lift your arm out in front of your body, this will tend to pull the vertebrae out of alignment because of the shift in center of gravity and the activity of muscle chains connecting the arm to the core. Therefore, the vertebrae need to be stabilized by core musculature in advance of the arm movement. But optimum stability does not prevent all movement in the spine — instead it allows small movements under control. Thus, proper stability, including core stability, is about a finely nuanced *control* of movement, as opposed to rigid *prevention* of movement.[6]

That is why graceful movements, even small subtle movements, affect the whole body. When a dancer lifts an arm, we do not see a rigid immobility of the core. Instead, we see subtle waves of compensatory movement through the core and the legs. Optimal stability is responsive, like the movement of a tree in the wind. In this sense, it is often more about subtle coordination and timing than brute strength.

Position: Joint Centration, Alignment, and Posture

It is interesting that we can usually recognize great movement from a static picture — which doesn't show actual movement! The reason the picture is revealing is that it shows relative joint positions, and position matters.

The position of a joint is a key determinant of its ability to function safely and effectively in a particular context. For example, it is safer to land a jump when the knees are aligned with the feet than when they are collapsed inward. It is safer to pick up heavy weight from the floor with the low back in neutral compared to rounded forward into full flexion. And the shoulder joint is far more capable of powerful and precise movement when the hands are extended in front of the body as opposed to behind.

When a particular joint is in optimal position for safety and performance with regard to a particular function, we can say the joint is in neutral, or centrated. Centration implies maximum bony contact between the two bones forming a joint, which allows the safest and most effective transfer of force. It also means that muscles will be at their optimal length for powerful coordinated movement.

When a series of adjacent joints are centrated for a common function, we can call this proper alignment, or posture. For example, if each vertebra is in relative neutral compared to its neighbor (not flexed, extended, rotated, or side bent) then the spine is in a well-aligned posture for many functions, including vertical loading.

Let's discuss these concepts in a little more detail.

Neutral joints create movement options

Moshe Feldenkrais stated that one of the most important criteria for good movement is the ability to move in any direction at any time with a minimum of preparation.

When a joint is in a neutral position, it has a full range of movement options. It can move forward or back, right or left with equal ease. When a joint is already in its end range of motion in a particular direction, it is strongly biased toward movement in the opposite direction, and there are fewer movement choices. It's like having your back against the wall in a game of tag.

Great movers have their joints in neutral as often as possible, preserving a full array of powerful movement options at any time. This is why static pictures of great athletes often reveal poise and balance.

Some common directions into which people tend to lose neutral joint position during movement are upper cervical extension, thoracic flexion, scapular elevation and internal rotation, thoracolumbar extension, hip flexion, and foot pronation.

Neutral joints absorb load and transfer force

When a joint absorbs a compressive load (e.g. the knee during a landing), a centrated position of the joint implies there is maximum contact between the ends of the two bones forming the joint. A broad area of contact distributes the load and prevents excessive stress in a small area. A narrow area of contact, for example a valgus (knock-knee) position, will tend to stress the lateral part of the bones and the medial ligaments. Small differences in joint angle can have large mechanical effects.

The angle between two bones will determine how well force is transferred between them. Bones are designed to push each other around. We can walk because the lower leg pushes into the femur, which pushes into the pelvis, which moves the center of gravity in the opposite direction of the angle of the push. Proper joint centration ensures that when one bone pushes into another, it goes in the intended direction. If the joint is not properly centrated, the push will cause random movements away from the intended pathway. They might also cause shearing, friction, excess mechanical stress in a local area, and the need for compensatory muscle activity.

Imagine the excellent feeling of hitting a golf ball or baseball right in the center. There is a perfect transfer of force from the club or bat into the ball. The ball moves away at maximum speed in a straight line with very little sense of effort or feeling of impact through your hands. By contrast, an off-center hit sends a horrible feeling of vibration through your hands and arms. The ball goes in an unpredictable direction, with minimal speed.

The same dynamics are at play in your joints when they accept a compressive load. If you push a heavy object such as a door, or punch a heavy bag, proper alignment of the wrist, elbow, shoulder joint, scapula, spine and hips, all the way down to the feet will ensure a clean transfer of force from the hand to the ground. The force passes *through* you. There are no energy leaks in the transmission which will create friction, shearing forces and other stresses that impair efficiency and cause microdamage. The same dynamics are at play each time we take a step.

In an erect posture, proper alignment of the bones allows the force of gravity to "pass through" the body to the ground cleanly. Just as blocks that are well stacked can resist gravity from pulling them down, bones that are well aligned can hold us up with only a minimum of muscular effort to maintain the alignment. Visualizing skeletal connections is an interesting way to simplify ideas about what movements are efficient.

Division of Labor

As stated before, movement is a team game with many players, in this case the muscles and joints. Let's examine the different kinds of work this team must perform, and how that work is optimally distributed.

Distribution of motion

Most movements are multisegmental — they involve movement at many joints in sequence. For example, if you bend to touch your toes, numerous joints will cooperate to move you in the desired direction.

If each joint contributes a moderate range of motion according to its own anatomy, then no one joint has to push beyond its comfortable range of motion. On the other hand, if for some reason one of the segments does not contribute much motion, then other joints will be obliged to push beyond their comfort zone. These joints will move farther away from a neutral position, which as we noted before is necessary to optimize power, balance, and control.

Take the simple example of turning to look behind you. You have twenty-four vertebrae in your spine, each of which are capable of some amount of rotation with respect to its neighbor (some more than others, of course). If the work of rotation is proportionately distributed amongst the vertebrae according to their rotational ability, then the movement will be experienced as smooth and easy. But if some of the vertebrae are not contributing to the movement, then others will be put under mechanical stress.

Good distribution of motion is actually pretty easy to see, even if we look from a distance. When we watch an elite performer moving through a large range of motion, say a pitch in baseball or an arabesque in dancing, we see proportional movement across many joints that is pleasing to the eye. You can trace a line from one foot, through to the pelvis, through the spine all the way to the opposite arm and find smooth, flowing, graceful arcs.

But if the motion is not well distributed throughout the body, you will see discontinuities: sharp angles followed by flat lines, an indication that some areas are working too hard, while others don't work at all. This is why Dr. Eric Cobb says we can identify efficient movement by looking for "arches not angles." It is interesting to consider that many years after the angled walls of an ancient building have fallen into ruin, an arched doorway will remain standing. The same is true in the body — sharp angles followed by flat lines is a sign of weakness, whereas smooth arches indicate strength.

Patterns of poor movement distribution

Many movement experts agree there are predictable patterns in the way people tend to deviate from an optimal division of labor with regard to range of motion. In other words, there are some areas that tend toward flat lines and others toward sharp angles.

Although there are various models to describe these patterns (Cook and Boyle's "joint by joint" model, Sahrmann's "directional susceptibility to movement," Janda's "upper and lower crossed" syndromes, McGill's "spinal hinge"), they are all based on at least two ideas.[7] First, excess stiffness at one joint will cause compensatory hypermobility at an adjacent joint that is a team member in the same multisegmental movement. Second, these patterns are to some extent predictable. Interestingly, the different models converge in their guesses on which areas are more likely to become facilitated in movement, and which are more likely to become stiff.

For example, the thoracic spine tends to become excessively stiff into extension and rotation, and the lumbar and cervical vertebrae compensate by becoming hypermobile into each of these directions. To use the team analogy, the thoracic spine is sitting on the bench during extension and rotation, while the low back and neck are doing extra work in the field and possibly getting injured as a result. For example, in an upward dog position, a common error might be too much extension in the low back and neck, and not enough in the upper back. It would be unusual to see the reverse.

Another common observation is that the hips tend toward stiffness into flexion, extension and rotation, which invites compensatory excess movement in the low back, knees or, subtalar joints. For example, in a forward bend movement, if the hips are too stiff, the low back moves into too much flexion to compensate. This is why so many different movement therapies recommend mobilizing the hips while at the same time stiffening the core. It is hard to think of any school of movement thought that recommends the opposite.

Distribution of work: power versus control

High quality movement also requires effective division of labor in regard to force production. The purpose of generating force through muscle contraction is to channel that force to a target, usually through the hands and feet. The most common target is the ground — the resulting ground reaction force is what moves our body around in locomotion.

The efficiency of this process depends on a good division of labor. Specifically, the big strong muscles should be doing the work of creating power, and the smaller more coordinated muscles should be doing the job of directing and channeling that power to its intended target.[8] To use the team analogy, this means making sure the coxswain is steering and the rowers are rowing, not vice versa.

The biggest strongest muscles are all located near the center of the body — the glutes, abdominals, hamstrings, quadriceps, hip flexors and spinal erectors. They are big and strong muscles because they need to move the pelvis, the largest bony mass in the body. Movement of the pelvis transfers forces to the shoulders and legs, which then move the hands and feet, which is where we usually interact with the environment.

The smaller muscles that connect the forearms to the hands and the lower leg to the foot are weaker, but more capable of very precise and controlled movements. As such, they are perfectly suited to channel forces very precisely to their final destination — such as the ground, a soccer ball, a baseball, or a punching bag.

This division of labor can get disturbed. If the strong prime mover muscles in the middle of the body are preoccupied with some task other than creating powerful movements (say in providing stability or balance), or for some reason inhibited in their function, then the smaller muscles might become obliged to become too involved in force production. This makes it harder for them to do their job of accurately channeling forces because brute force exertion prevents a finely nuanced control.

This dynamic explains why we repeatedly hear from various sports or martial arts experts that powerful movement should be initiated or generated from the center of the body, or the core, or the pelvis, or the dantien. The importance of the pelvis for power generation is easy to miss when watching great athletes or dancers, because our attention tends to be drawn to the periphery of the body, where skillful and intricate gestures are made at high speed. But these movements originate in the center. The amazing hand speed generated by an elite golfer or baseball player starts with a powerful translation and rotation of the hips.

Another common issue with distribution of work occurs when muscles that are better suited for local segmental stability become inhibited, while the muscles better suited for global stability and large movement become facilitated. We will discuss this specific issue in more detail later in the book.

Good Movement is Efficient

We can think of great movement as offering the most *benefit* in terms of achieving functional objectives, at the least *cost* to the body in terms of energy or physical stress. In this sense, it is efficient. We can define efficiency in movement as the ratio of useful work performed compared to the cost (either in energy or mechanical stress) required to perform it.

One of the main impressions you will receive from watching an elite athlete or dancer is that what they are doing looks incredibly easy. Imagine a gymnast performing a back flip, a shortstop fielding a ground ball and firing to first, or a skier slaloming around poles. These are all powerful moves that accomplish a great deal of work, but because they are performed with such efficiency, they can be done for hundreds of repetitions without fatigue or injury.

By contrast, if the same movements were performed by a person without a high level of skill, *even a person with great fitness,* that person would be exhausted or injured after only a few repetitions.

Professional marathon runners use about 30 percent less energy to accomplish the same work as an average runner. Their movement is so fluid they look like perpetual motion machines or a ball rolling downhill. By contrast, many runners look more like rolling triangles. Each step is costly in terms of energy and mechanical stress.

Many runners think running faster is all about getting fitter and better able to expend energy. They want to put a bigger engine in the car. That is a good idea of course, but another key factor in performance is simply learning to take the foot off the brake. Driving with the brake means you don't go anywhere very fast and you damage your car in the process. Similarly, inefficient movement can slow you down and stress the body at the same time.

The Skill of Relaxation

Efficient movement requires skill in relaxation. For example, in sprinting, any muscle that contracts to push you forward will be asked to relax and lengthen in the next phase of the gait cycle. If the muscle is slow to lengthen, it essentially put the brakes on forward movement. For these reasons, world-famous sprint coach Charlie Francis considered relaxation to be the number one secret to greater speed. Even if relaxing means you generate less absolute force, it may result in an increase in the net force pushing you forward.[9]

Golfers, tennis players, and baseball pitchers would give similar advice about executing maximum power. Some element of relaxation is always necessary during maximum speed, and working too hard has the unintended effect of slowing you down. Again, this is why great athletes make it look easy, generating enormous power even while looking very relaxed and smooth.

Relaxation skill is also important to prevent excess muscular tension in everyday life. A person working at a computer needs to move only his fingers and wrists. However, the stress of the work will often cause what Moshe Feldenkrais called parasitic tension — unwanted and unnecessary muscle contractions in many other areas (e.g. the shoulders, neck, or jaw). We could make similar observations about other activities we do all day long such as reaching, breathing, walking, sitting or standing. Excess tension in these activities is unlikely to cause any discomfort over the course of a minute or two, but accumulated over the course of days, weeks and years, the effects may become significant.

In general, inhibition of muscular activity is a higher order skill than activation, which tends to spread or irradiate from place to place without any help. Put another way, it is relatively easy to activate a muscle — the hard thing is keeping it relaxed when its neighbors are working.

Imagine playing the piano. Each time you activate the muscles of one finger to strike a key, you must relax all the others so the wrong key isn't struck at the same time. The inhibition is more important than the activation.

An infant has almost no ability to control the spread of muscular excitement from one place to another. Any intention to accomplish a local movement goal tends to activate all the muscles in the body. Reaching for an object gets the legs kicking.

Similarly, when a novice tries to perform a complex activity for the first time, almost every muscle becomes involved in the movement. Salsa dancing will create excess tension in the hands and arms. A golf swing will activate the facial muscles.

Part of the reason this occurs is that a novice learning a new skill will simplify the complexity of the movement by locking certain joints into place. This effectively reduces the moving parts and variables associated with movement, making motor control easier.[10] But this strategy also requires sustained and excess muscle tension, which is less efficient. And by locking certain joints into place, it fails to take advantage of potential "team members" whose movements can assist with power and control.

Moving from novice to expert implies releasing degrees of freedom at the joints through relaxation of muscular tension. For example, a novice basketball player learning to dribble will simplify the interaction of the shoulder, elbow and wrist in performing the movement by essentially locking the elbow in place. As skill is gained, movement at the elbow is incorporated. Just as moving from a tricycle to a bicycle requires control of more variables, but provides more power, efficiency and accuracy, moving from the use of two joints to three provides similar advantages in dribbling a basketball.[11]

Thus, developing movement skill is often more about learning to inhibit the spread of neural excitement rather than extending it. In this sense, *learning better movement is more like sculpture than painting*. You improve your art by taking things away, not adding them.

Rhythm and Timing

Optimum coordination requires the right muscles to fire at the right *time* and the joints to move in the proper *sequence*. Although correct timing of muscle activation is often unique to the particular situation, there are at least a few general rules about timing that apply to almost all examples of quality movement.

One requirement, as noted earlier, is that stability muscles fire *before* the prime movers. Interestingly, as we will see in a later section, there is significant research showing this timing can be disturbed in people with chronic pain.

Proper timing is also necessary to ensure muscles contract at their optimum length. Most muscles will fire most efficiently and powerfully if they are preloaded into a moderate stretch before contracting. This allows the muscle to take advantage of elastic recoil and stretch reflexes. During most functional movements, entire chains of muscle are lengthened and shortened in sequence. Walking or running is a perfect example of this pattern of activity — limbs go back before going forward, and muscles lengthen before shortening. Proper timing in this sense manifests as a smooth and flowing wave of movement through the body that is easy to see and pleasing to the eye.

Here's an experiment to feel how waiting for a muscle to be pre-stretched will make its contraction more reflexive, automatic and easy. During walking, imagine your trailing leg is like a rag doll with no muscles. Relax it as much as possible. Keep the trailing foot on the ground as long as possible, until forward movement of the pelvis stretches the hip flexors far enough so they drag the leg forward passively. You will feel that the trailing leg moves forward quickly and easily without any feeling of effort or even conscious intention to move it. This is because you have taken full advantage of the elastic properties of the hip flexors and quads, and their activation has been more reflexive than deliberate. You can notice something similar while walking up stairs. As you step up with the right foot, think about putting your full weight onto the foot. You may feel your left foot lifting from the floor to move upward even without intending to lift it. The movement of the rest of the body forward pulls the left leg along to join it.

The golf swing is another good example. The first thing that happens on the downswing is the pelvis rotates and translates toward the target. The movement of the pelvis pulls on the abs, which then pull on the rib cage and spine, causing each to rotate to the target. The rib cage then pulls the scapula, which pulls the upper arm to the target. Then the right elbow extends. Only then does the right wrist, the weakest, but most precise link in the chain finally release into impact. Each of these joint movements happens in a flowing, rhythmic sequence. Each successive lever in the movement chain is weaker and smaller, but is moving faster and is more coordinated. If a joint moves out of turn (such as "coming over the top" by moving the arms before the rib cage) then power is leaked and accuracy is compromised. Similar wave-like sequential movements can be seen in other powerful movements such as kicking, punching, throwing, or sprinting.

Optimal timing and rhythm depend on the individual. Everybody has muscles and connective tissues of different lengths and elasticities. Therefore, for each given structure, there is an optimal rhythm for large amplitude synergistic movements.

People with short limbs and thick muscles, like Mike Tyson or Barry Sanders, will move in characteristically short, choppy, piston-like movements. People with longer limbs and thinner muscle bellies will start their movements fairly slowly but then crack their bodies like whips as forces are slowly summated. Think of a long lanky pitcher slowly building speed.

An athlete's ability to feel and maintain the unique rhythm of their particular body is an important determinant of the quality of their movement. This is particularly obvious in running, sprinting, throwing and other large amplitude of whole body movements that involve sequenced rhythmic timing of muscle chains.

Balance

Balance is the ability to maintain center of gravity within the base of support. Great movers of course have great balance.

Humans are unique in the animal kingdom in that they have a very small base of support and a very high center of gravity. Moshe Feldenkrais made the interesting observation that statues of humans need to be built with a very heavy and wide base to prevent them from toppling over. By contrast, a statue of an animal on four legs is stable without external assistance.

The same features that make humans relatively unstable in a standing position also provide them with greater stored potential energy to move in any direction with very little hesitation. In other words, a person who is standing up can do a lot of the work of moving in any particular direction by simply allowing their body to fall in that direction. Think of a sprinter falling forward to start a race.

Great balance is not just about staying upright while walking a balance beam. Even in situations where falling is not a threat, optimal balance is required to preserve the ability to move in any direction with a minimum of preparation. If your center of gravity is leaning too far to one side, you've lost the ability to move quickly to the other side. In sports, that can be the difference between winning and losing. In dance or gymnastics, it can be the break in rhythm that ruins a routine.

An interesting way to test the quality of your balance at any particular point on a movement path is to see if you can change your direction, even in the opposite direction. In this sense, "reversibility" is sometimes a good test of movement quality.

One aspect of balance that accounts for some of the aesthetically pleasing aspects of good movement is counterbalance. Given that humans have such a small base of support, any significant movement of an arm or leg will tend to bring the center of gravity outside the base of support in that direction. Therefore, to maintain the center of gravity over the base of support, another limb has to be moved in an equal and opposite direction. If you take a snapshot of any elite mover in action, you'll see a beautiful example of reciprocal use of the limbs for counterbalance. A dancer performing an arabesque, or a soccer player kicking a ball are perfect examples. We actually see this counterbalance in every step we take — when the right leg moves forward, the left leg moves back, etc. It is another indication that even distant parts of the body are functionally related.

Responsiveness and Variability

Good movement is not just about harmonious interaction or coordination between the different parts of the body. It is most fundamentally about how the system interacts with the environment, particularly in response to unexpected changes. In other words, good movement implies a quality of adaptability and responsiveness to a changing environment.[12]

One can imagine building a humanoid robot that can walk with flawless symmetry and grace. But if the robot cannot *adapt* its gait pattern to accommodate changes in the terrain, it will fall each time it steps on a rock, and its movement skill is essentially useless. True movement intelligence therefore doesn't exist so much in the movements themselves, but in their interaction with the environment.

The graceful stride of the deer isn't useful unless it can be modulated to jump a log and avoid a wolf. A soccer player who can execute technically brilliant ball handling skills in solo practice does not face the real test until she performs those moves in a game situation, spontaneously, against an opponent who is actively trying to disrupt her.

We would not say that someone is fluent in a language if they have only one way to communicate a particular thought, regardless of how perfect that particular communication is. Similarly, one is not fluent in the language of movement unless he can accomplish the same goal in many different ways.

A person who can move from standing to sitting with perfect smoothness, but through only one particular trajectory, has less resourcefulness than someone who can modulate their descent to the floor in many ways. The power lifter who can perform a squat with perfect form is not necessarily prepared for a day of gardening, where the squatting movements need to constantly adapt to the environment — slightly off center, with the feet in different positions. (To be fair, the gardener is probably not prepared to squat 800 pounds either.) Thus, we cannot always measure good movement by its adherence to some ideal form, but rather in its capacity to adapt to many different situations.

This capacity for adaptability and resourcefulness does not apply only to competitive sports. Our everyday lives constantly present unexpected movement or postural challenges. A long plane ride in a cramped seat. A night on the couch or in a strange bed. Walking in shoes that are uncomfortable. Carrying groceries in one hand while loading a baby into a car. In each of these situations, solving the motor problem might require a departure from what is normally considered "good" posture, proper form, or the most beautifully harmonious way to move. The ability to find a motor solution to all these unexpected problems is part of what we should consider to be motor intelligence.

Good Movement Feels Good

Sitting with "perfect posture" or running with impeccable gait, or downward dogging just like the yoga teacher isn't good movement if it doesn't *feel* good — painless, comfortable, authentic and effortless. This should go without saying, but it can be easy to forget.

We spend a lot of time moving in a way that will conform to the social norms of body language, or win a sports trophy, or look good to a dance audience, or please personal trainers, yoga instructors or physical therapists who tell us the "right" way to move. Many people try to arrange their posture in accordance with the advice of some expert, even though it doesn't feel natural or comfortable. And many other people simply ignore the feedback from their body altogether, until it is hard for them to even know whether a particular area is in pain. The result is a loss of sensitivity to information from the body that could help us determine the "rightness" of a particular movement or posture, and then make intelligent adjustments.

As we age, it is easy to forget what it feels like for certain movements to be completely comfortable. If you have lived past the age of thirty, there are probably several movements you do regularly that create at least some minor amount of discomfort each time you do them. Perhaps squatting to pick something up off the floor, reaching overhead, or looking behind you to back out of a parking space. The failure to perceive the discomfort makes it impossible to work for, or even imagine improvements that may be quite achievable.

Another subtle indication of the "rightness" of a particular movement that people often ignore is whether it feels natural, authentic and effortless. Most of us have experienced the excellent feeling of suddenly correcting a movement in a way that made it feel far easier. This often occurs in the context of learning a sport or novel activity. What formerly felt awkward and wrong suddenly feels natural and right. In the context of everyday life, many people have significant room for improvement in how natural and easy they breathe, rise from a chair, or move their pelvis. Developing a more subtle appreciation for differences in this regard is an important component of learning better movement.

Individual

Good movement is individual. Although I definitely believe there are certain general rules for good movement (that's the whole point of this chapter!) I should also point out that they don't apply to everyone.

Everyone has a different structure and therefore the optimal movement solution for one person will not be the same as for another. This is particularly true in the case of joint centration, posture and alignment. Good posture for someone with scoliosis is not the same as good posture for someone without. Asking someone with scoliosis to stand with their vertebrae in a straight line is basically asking them to move their vertebrae *away* from neutral positions.

Further, many people have a bony structure that prevents them from centrating all their joints at the same time in regard to a particular function. If you have a tibial torsion, where the bottom of the tibia rotates internally with respect to the upper part, you may not be able to have your hip, knee and ankle centrated at the same time while squatting. For this person, finding a movement solution to squatting or other activities might very well imply deviations from what is commonly considered to be good form.

Posture

Posture refers to the orientation of the body or the spine when not a lot of gross movement is occurring, as in sitting, standing, or otherwise waiting for something else to happen. Posture is really just another form of movement — it takes skilled and coordinated work of the muscles and proper positioning and alignment of the joints. Further, posture always involves some small degree of movement — breathing, oscillations around a center point, turning the head from side to side, etc.

Because the quality of posture is determined by the quality of the muscular organization required to sustain it, we can judge posture by applying the same principles used to define good movement. Thus, just like movement, good posture is efficient, relaxed, coordinated, aligned, and involves a proper division of labor between postural and prime mover muscles.

Good posture maintains joints in a neutral position that allows an easy transition to the maximum amount of useful movements with a minimum of preparation. Good posture feels good and effortless. Good posture is also responsive to the environment and depends on the needs of the moment. Therefore, good sitting posture is different when you are typing, watching TV, eating dinner, or driving a car.

Posture is individual to each person and depends on their particular structure. Posture benefits from having a large assortment of options to solve the problem of how to just hang out and do nothing.

In short, posture is a dynamic thing whose quality is judged in terms of its ability to facilitate meaningful interactions with the environment, and not its conformance to an abstract ideal or plumb line.

Surprisingly, and in marked contrast to the claims of many people who tout "bad" posture as being the cause of many chronic pain conditions, most studies looking at measurable differences in posture between individuals find that such differences do not predict differences in chronic pain levels.[13]

This should be a very strong caution to anyone trying to explain pain in relation to postural deviation from the norm. However, these caveats do not imply that posture does not matter for function. Optimal coordination of the limbs absolutely requires optimal coordination and alignment of the spine as a foundation. As stated by noted Russian physiologist Nikolai Bernstein, trying to move with poor posture is like trying to write with a floppy pencil.

Summary

Here is a brief summary of the major points in this chapter, followed by some caveats and limitations to keep in mind.

Movement that is biomechanically efficient, functional and healthy is characterized by the following general qualities:

* *Coordination:* Movement is a team game, and proper teamwork between the joints and muscles is more important than their individual performance.

* *Responsiveness:* No matter how coordinated movement is, it is useless if it cannot respond to changes and variations in the environment.

* *Distribution of effort:* The mechanical stress of movement needs to be distributed over as many team members as possible. The more team members involved in performing the work of movement, the more work can be done. Multisegmental movements should create proportional and distributed arcs, as opposed to angles.

* *Division of labor:* Muscles should perform the role to which they are best suited: stabilizers stabilize, prime movers move, large muscles create power, smaller muscles direct forces.

* *Position and alignment:* Joints are safest and most functional when they are in a neutral or centrated position. Coordinated movement keeps joints centrated and aligned as often as possible.

* *Relaxation and efficiency:* Movement skill is characterized by inhibition of unnecessary muscular work and parasitic tension. Inhibition is a higher-order skill than activation.

* *Timing:* Stabilizer muscles need to fire before prime movers. Multi-segmental movements require proper sequencing. Most movements require that muscles lengthen before shortening to take advantage of elastic recoil, the passive properties of the soft tissues, and reflexive muscle activation.

* *Variability:* Movement is like a language. Fluency is judged by variability not just precision.

* *Comfort:* Movement should be pain free, effortless, and natural.

* *Individual:* Optimal movement solutions are always customized to fit the individual, task and environment.

The lessons at the end of this book are intended to teach students to gain better awareness and control over all these qualities of movement.

Caveats

Following are some caveats to keep in mind in regard to the material presented in this chapter:

* The above criteria for good movement are not intended to replace criteria based on precise objective measurement that are specific to a particular joint or movement. Instead, they are to provide insights that can be missed with an approach that is heavily reliant on measurements that might be inaccurate or biomechanical assumptions that might be incorrect.

* Not everyone can learn to move like a professional athlete or dancer just by studying or applying these principles! Although great movement is

very much about *skill*, it's also about the *structure* of the body. A 1972 Pinto cannot be driven as well as a Ferrari, no matter how expert the driver. We should not compare ourselves to the unusual people on the playing field or stage who were born with optimal structures for the activity they are performing. Thus, if our movement is not perfect according to the above principles, it does not imply that our movement skills are to blame. (With that being said, most people have room for improvement!)

* If movement is a skill that can be improved, it is also a habit that can be hard to break. Some changes are easy to make, but others require real effort. We will discuss this idea in the chapter on motor control.

* Perfect biomechanics do not guarantee being pain-free. As we will discuss in the section on pain, it is often driven by factors that have little to do with tissue damage caused by the stress of movement. Thus, one can have apparently perfect movement in a certain area and still suffer pain, and vice versa. Nevertheless, the way we move is definitely one form of stress on the body, and we would rather have less than more!

CHAPTER 2

LEARNING BETTER MOVEMENT

"Much more of the brain is devoted to movement than to language. Language is only a little thing sitting on top of this huge ocean of movement."
— Oliver Sacks

HOW DO WE IMPROVE skill in movement? In this chapter, we will look at how the nervous system perceives and controls the movement of the body, and how it can learn to perform these functions better.

Controlling the movement of a human body is an amazing accomplishment of engineering and information processing. It is easy to underestimate the challenge, because most of the work is unconscious.

As we walk or do almost anything, there are millions of bits of information about joint and muscle position flowing from the body to the brain. This information has to be assembled and processed into a meaningful understanding of where everything is and what it is doing. And there are millions of muscle fibers that need to be told how to contract or relax in order to create a coordinated movement. All of this occurs beneath our conscious awareness.

The degree of information processing required to accomplish this task is staggering. It is the rough equivalent of controlling a puppet with millions of strings attached to millions of contractile elements that control hundreds of joints that can all move through many degrees of freedom. The brain's accomplishments in regard to controlling movement are in many ways more impressive than its abstract reasoning abilities.

For example, we have created a computer program that can beat the world's greatest chess players, but cannot build a robot that can load a dishwasher. Computers can compose credible symphonies, destroy Jeopardy champions, and carry on conversations that seem very human. But no robot can even come close to the movement skill of a three year old in walking from place to place, picking up objects, and performing other simple movements we completely take for granted.

In this chapter we will look at the hardware and software that allows us to solve movement problems. This will help us understand how we can change the software to create better outcomes in the way we move and feel.

The Elements of Motor Control

Motor control is the process by which we organize and execute our movements. We can divide the motor control system into three separate subsystems: passive, active and neural.[14] The first two comprise the "hardware" that moves us around, while the third is the "software" that gathers information, interprets it, and issues commands. Here's a brief description of the three subsystems and how they cooperate to provide motor control.

The Active System: Muscle Contraction

The active system is comprised of the muscles. Each muscle has many thousands of muscle fibers, which are grouped together into motor units. A motor unit fires on an all or nothing basis — either all the muscle fibers in the unit fire, or none fire. Large muscles generally have more fibers per unit than smaller muscles. For example, the muscles controlling the fingers have only 350 fibers per unit, whereas the muscles in the thigh have about 1000 muscle fibers per unit. This means the fingers have far more precise control over force production than the knees.

Muscle fibers work by creating tension. As tension is created, the length of the fiber may shorten (a concentric contraction), lengthen (eccentric contraction), or remain the same length (isometric contraction). For example, in a dumb-bell curl, the biceps contracts concentrically to lift the weight, isometrically to prevent the weight from dropping during a pause, and eccentrically to control the lowering of the weight.

Because the muscle fibers are the only active players in the movement system, we can think of any movement as being completely defined by a certain pattern of activity of the motor units. In other words, making a certain movement is simply a matter of activating the right motor units at the right time, at the right length, in the right sequence.

The Passive System: Connective Tissue

The passive subsystem is comprised of all the movement hardware aside from the muscles — the bones, joint capsules, cartilage, fascia, tendons, ligaments and other connective tissues (also the passive properties of the muscles). The passive system does a great deal of the work of movement without the expenditure of any energy.

For example, each time you move your body weight over your stance foot during walking, the achilles tendon stretches to store elastic energy, and then returns some of this energy in the form of a propulsive force. Learning to move with efficiency is characterized by making greater use of the passive system to perform work.

Another way the passive system does work "for free" is by creating stability through passive restraints to movement. For example, if I lower my head to look at my toes, I could hold it there in two ways. I could create tension in the muscles at the back of my neck, or I could let those muscles relax so the head hangs passively from the soft tissues.

Imagine the posture of a slouching bored teenager — one hip kicked out to the side, hyperextended knees, collapsed chest and forward head position. In this position they are creating postural stability by basically hanging off the passive system, as opposed to actively working the muscles to keep the joints centrated and aligned. This strategy for creating stability is energetically cheap, but mechanically expensive in terms of the stress it places on the soft tissues in the passive system. It is also expensive in terms of being poorly prepared to transition into the next movement.

The passive system also does some of the work of controlling movement that would otherwise need to be performed by the neural system. This is done by limiting the degrees of freedom through which a joint can move, so that movement occurs on a predetermined path, as opposed to a path that needs to be chosen by intelligent decision-making and movement commands.

For example, the ankle has more passive restraints to movement and less degrees of freedom than the shoulder, and therefore requires far less muscle and brainpower to move through a desired pathway. If we rely too much on the passive system to determine the pathways through which we move, like the slouching teenager, this reduces the burden on the neural and muscular systems to control movement, but again places excess stress on the passive system.

The Nervous System: Information Processing

The nervous system's function in motor control can be thought of as an information processing machine.[15] The peripheral nervous system gathers inputs — information about the health, position and movement of the body parts. The central nervous system processes this information and creates two basic outputs — conscious perceptions about the body, and motor commands to move the body.

Following is a discussion of several basic key concepts relating to the nervous system's control of movement, including sensation, perception, and the production of motor commands.

Sensation — gathering information

Sensation is the process by which the body detects a stimulus and sends a signal toward the brain. (As we'll discuss in the next section, sensation is a distinct concept from perception.)[16]

Numerous sensors within the body can help the brain detect the position and movement of the different body parts. Of primary importance is information coming from the proprioceptive, visual and vestibular systems.

The proprioceptive system provides information from the mechanoreceptors, which are located in skin, joints, connective tissue, ligaments, tendons, and muscles. The mechanoreceptors have various names such as ruffinis, meisner corpuscles, pacinian corpuscles, golgi tendon organs, and muscle spindle fibers. Each of them responds to a different type of mechanical stimulus. Some respond to stretch, others to pressure, some to quick movements, others to sustained movements. When they are triggered, they send a signal to the central nervous system indicating that something is happening. For example, the sensor might report that a ligament is stretching, a joint is being compressed, a muscle is lengthening, or the skin is stretching.[17]

Vision provides important information about the body's orientation in space and its relation to the environment. Without vision, body sense is significantly compromised, and this is why you will find it harder to balance on one foot with your eyes closed.

The vestibular system provides information about the movement of the head and its orientation relative to the line of gravity. Without it, we can barely stand up. Part of the reason drunk people have poor balance is that alcohol compromises the vestibular system.

Perception — interpreting sensory information

Although the terms sensation and perception are often used interchangeably in everyday life, psychologists distinguish between them. The distinction is very useful in understanding movement.

Sensation is the detection of a stimulus and the transmission of a signal toward the central nervous system. Perception is the process of taking that sensory information, filtering it, organizing it, and interpreting its meaning to create a subjective or conscious experience related to the sensation.[18]

For example, through sensation the ears report information about sound waves to the brain, and through perception we hear music. In the context of movement, sensation reports proprioceptive and vestibular information, and perception creates a felt sense of the movement.

It is useful to distinguish between the two because they are not identical. Many factors can modulate perception, including the way we focus our attention, our past experience, and our expectations. Thus, two people can receive the same sensory information, but perceive completely different things.

Look at the picture below:

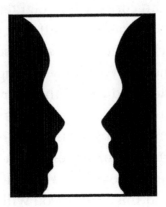

You can "see" it in two different ways — as one vase, or two faces looking at each other. The sensory data flowing from the eyes remains the same, but the perception of the picture completely changes as the brain alternates back and forth between competing interpretations of what the data means. Notice that you can't "see" both pictures at the same time!

The illusion reveals there is a great degree of nearly instantaneous calculation and interpretation happening beneath our awareness, before we see anything. Our experience of vision is not a pure reflection of the real world — it is our brain's *construction* of a picture that it thinks is a useful representation of what we need to know about the world.

Here's another fun illusion to make this point a little more clear. Look at the picture of the chessboard. It looks like squares A and B are different colors right?

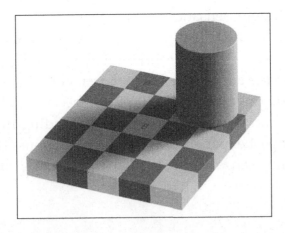

But they're not! You can see they are the same color when a band is drawn between them.

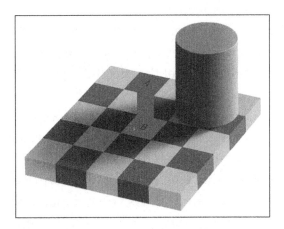

Now I bet you are thinking the pictures are somehow rigged, but you can put a finger over the band between the squares and watch them transform back into different colors. (I've done this myself many times!)

Why do the colors on A and B look different? Your brain creates this perception because it takes into account the effect of the shadow cast by the cylinder, and the alternating pattern of the squares. Based on this information, it guesses that the apparent sameness of the colors is actually a trick of the light. So it makes them look different. It is absolutely amazing how much intelligent decision-making is going on at lightning speed beneath our conscious awareness. We never "see" the raw data — we only perceive pictures that our brain constructs, which it thinks will best serve our needs.

Similarly, our kinesthetic sense of the body is not just a mirror of body position, but a construction that is created to serve functional goals. Just as you can see the same picture different ways, you can perceive the same movement in different ways, depending on how you interpret the sense data created by the movement.

We know this because as you get better at a particular activity, your perception of body position will change significantly, even as the sensory information associated with the movement remains the same. Imagine performing a complex movement for the first time, such as a backflip, a new dance move, or a golf swing. Your perceptions about the position of your body during the movement will probably be confused. In other words, you literally won't know what you are doing, and you won't be able to predict the consequences of your movements.

This is not because of some defect in sensation, or the quality of proprioceptive information flowing to the brain. The problem is in perception — the nervous system's ability to interpret the meaning of the sensory information. In the case of a novel movement, the brain has no past experience organizing similar information, and therefore it does a poor job.[19]

With practice, the brain gets feedback about the correspondence between a particular perception and actual reality. For example, if you perceive that your feet are in good position to land a flip, you will quickly realize your mistake when you land on your butt. As you get more feedback, perception about body position will improve, and eventually you will know where everything is and what it is doing during the movement.

Therefore, the difference between an elite athlete and an everyday Joe in terms of body sense is probably more about perception than sensation. Each is likely receiving similar sensory information about movement, but the athlete has far more skill in accurately and quickly interpreting the meaning of that information and creating functionally useful perceptions.

Motor commands — the key output

The whole point of collecting sensory information and forming perceptions about body position is to help decide what motor commands will produce useful movements.

If you think about it from an evolutionary perspective, the only real purpose for *any* mental activity is to assist making the right movements: moving the body toward food and shelter, and away from predators; manipulating tools; moving the mouth and vocal cords in a way that communicates ideas to friends and family.

An interesting illustration of the uselessness of a brain in a body without movement is the sea squirt, which spends the first part of its life as an animal moving around, and the second part attaching itself to a rock and then camping out as a plant. As soon as it settles down, does it use this time as an opportunity to meditate or think about the meaning of life? No, it eats its brain for the energy. This should make use very curious about what happens to a human brain in a body that spends too much time on the couch.

Where do motor commands come from?

Motor commands originate from different levels of the nervous system — the spinal cord, the lower levels of the brain, and the higher levels of the brain. Motor commands that originate from higher centers in the brain can be modified as they descend by sensory signals arriving at the spinal cord level.[20] The level from which the motor command originates will be associated with whether the motor command is more in the nature of a reflex or more like a conscious decision.

On the reflexive end of the spectrum are movements like withdrawing a hand from a hot stove or maintaining balance in response to perturbation. In these cases, a stimulus from the periphery sends a signal to the spinal cord, and the spinal cord issues a motor command in response. Speed is the priority, so there is no time to allow the sensory signals to travel all the way to the brain for sophisticated analysis before movement commands are given. Because the movement happens before the stimulus is perceived, it feels effortless and involuntary. We make an enormous number of reflexive stabilizing muscle contractions each second to maintain an upright posture. Of course, we are usually not aware of any of them.

On the other end of the spectrum are complex multi-step movements like reaching for a wine glass over a crowded table, or threading a needle. After the movement starts, the brain looks to sensory feedback to monitor progress and make adjustments. This is called "closed loop" or feedback motor control, and it requires conscious attention and planning.[21]

The disadvantage of this type of motor control is that it is slow and incapable of multitasking. Try writing two different words simultaneously with your right and left hand. It's too tough because each movement requires attention. Closed loop motor control is therefore useless in circumstances where many things need to happen at once, or where there isn't enough time to process feedback during the movement and make adjustments.

For example, imagine swinging at a baseball pitch. This requires a sequence of motor commands to accomplish the swing. The hips must rotate toward the target, then the shoulders, then the arms extend, etc. But the swing needs to be completed before there is time for the brain to make adjustments in between the steps. Therefore, all the high-level commands that execute the different steps in the movement must be issued in advance. This is called open loop motor control or feed forward movement, and it is governed by a motor program.[22]

The program is built through a process of motor learning. In the novice stage, executing a series of coordinated motor commands requires significant conscious control and widespread brain activity in the cortex. But with more practice, the movement is controlled by more focused neural activity in the lower centers of the brain. The movement becomes more automatic, efficient and quick. And it causes far less interference with other ongoing activities, like walking, thinking or talking.

This is why when we start learning to drive, we have to pay very close attention to where our foot goes, where the hands go to shift, etc. Once we build a dedicated program to execute the skill, we are free to simultaneously perform other activities like tuning the radio or enjoying a delicious beverage. What a great thing!

Thus, we can see that motor commands that are more reflexive or automatic have several advantages — they are quick, efficient, and allow multitasking. Their disadvantage is being stereotyped, formulaic, and less responsive to novel changes in the environment. Motor commands originating from the higher centers of the brain have the opposite set of advantages and disadvantages.[23]

In many ways, gaining skill at a particular task involves making its performance more automated and efficient, and transferring responsibility for the movement from higher centers to lower centers. On the other hand, motor development during infancy is a process whereby the higher centers inhibit primitive reflexes from the lower areas, so that more differentiated responses to stimuli are possible. To complicate matters further, motor commands that originate in the brain from learned programs are modified by the incoming sensory information at the spinal cord level, so they are more responsive to changing conditions in the environment.

If this sounds confusing then you are getting my point. The intelligence responsible for motor control is widely distributed throughout the central nervous system from the spinal cord to the higher centers of the brain. The interactions between the different levels can be hierarchical and sequential, or parallel and simultaneous. The nature of these interactions is above all *complex*: like an ecosystem or market economy, the source of order is not centralized in any particular area, but *emerges* from the relatively simple interactions of trillions of different moving parts.[24]

Given this level of complexity, it is a good idea to look for a perspective that makes things simpler! If we try to understand the intelligence of the system by studying each individual part of the whole, it is easy to get lost. For example, we can learn about the myotactic stretch reflex, the function of the cerebellum, its interaction with the motor cortex. This might be very interesting and useful, but it leaves out the relevant contributions of thousands of other moving parts in the machine, many of which would require years of study to understand, and even more of which we probably don't know anything about anyway.

Therefore, looking at the nervous system from the perspective of the micro-level and the interaction of different parts might make it harder to see the big picture. We don't seek to understand the meaning of a movie by looking at the individual pixels of color on the screen. Similarly, it is easier to understand how the nervous system controls movement by looking at a higher level of abstraction.

The cortical maps provide a useful "big picture" that can simplify some of the complexity of motor control, because in many ways they are an objective representation of the intelligence of the entire system. We will take a look at the maps in the next chapter.

Before doing that, here is a brief summary of what we discussed in this chapter.

Summary

* Controlling a body with many degrees of freedom is one of the most amazing accomplishments of the brain.

* The motor control system can be thought of as an information processing machine. The inputs into the machine are bits of sensory information

from the body. The outputs are perceptions about body movement and motor commands to create movement. We are unaware of the amazing intelligence of this process because it is almost completely unconscious and instantaneous.

* Sensation is the process of collecting raw sensory data from the body, whether visual, vestibular, proprioceptive, or interoceptive.

* Perception is the process by which sensory data is interpreted and assigned meaning to create conscious or subjective experience that serves functional goals. Unlike sensation, perception is a skill that improves with practice.

* Motor control is incredibly complex, and emerges from the parallel and hierarchical interactions between different levels of the nervous system: the spinal cord, the subcortical areas of the brain, and the cortex.

CHAPTER 3

THE BRAIN MAPS THE BODY

"Everywhere you look in the brain, maps abound."
— V.S. Ramachandran

ONE OF THE MOST FASCINATING discoveries in modern neuroscience is that our conscious experience is created by patterns of brain activity. These patterns are often called maps.

Every thought, every emotion, every intention is the product of the brain's physical state. If someone could open your head and stimulate the pattern of brain activity associated with eating chocolate, or getting stung by a bee, or moving a finger, you would experience those events like they were really happening. Thus, when you consciously perceive the position or movement of a particular body part, there is a particular pattern of brain activity that creates the perception.[25]

The neurons that perceive the body and issue motor commands are often grouped together in discrete areas. For example, there is a part of your brain that is primarily devoted to perceiving your middle finger. This area becomes active whenever it receives sensory information from the finger. Further, if this area of your brain was somehow stimulated artificially, you would feel like you were being touched on the finger.

Similarly, if you decided to move your middle finger, a certain part of your brain would activate to issue the motor commands to do that. And, and if this part of your brain was artificially stimulated, your middle finger would move.[26]

The discrete parts of the brain that are devoted to moving or perceiving a particular body part are called cortical maps or body maps. They are also sometimes called sensory motor maps, the cortical body matrix or the body schema.

The relatively recent discovery of these maps is a very important advancement in our understanding of how we perceive and move the body. For example, the body maps help solve the riddle of a phantom limb — the uncannily real feeling that an amputated missing limb is actually still there. Even though the limb is gone, the maps that create the *feeling* of the limb are still intact and can be activated.[27] As stated by pain scientist Ronald Melzack, "We don't need a body to feel a body." All we need is stimulation of the body maps. This is a key insight. If body perception depends on the maps, the state of the map has huge implications for how we move and feel.

Neuroplasticity: the maps can change

One extremely interesting property of these maps is they change their shape, size and organization over time, and these changes correlate with changes in the way we move and perceive the body.

The ability of the brain to change is called neuroplasticity. This is a revolutionary concept that only recently overturned the previous belief that the organization of the brain was relatively fixed over time. We now know the brain is always adapting its anatomy and physiology to meet functional demands.

Researchers study neuroplasticity by measuring the size and activity of the cortical maps, and seeing how they change under certain conditions. Measurements are performed through various techniques like functional magnetic resonance imaging or microelectrodes. This allows researchers to track changes in the brain over time, as well as any associated changes in behavior. This research can provide significant insight into how we can change the brain to move better and feel better. For example, how does the brain change in response to injury, practice of a physical skill, or chronic pain? We now have quite a bit of research on these questions. Let's take a look.

Good Movement Requires a Good Map

The quality of movement and perception in a particular body part is determined in part by the size and quality of the motor sensory maps for that body part. If you have a very detailed map of a certain area, you can perceive and move that area with precision. If the map is less defined or "fuzzy," perception and movement will be less accurate.

We know this because body parts with greater movement and perception demands have bigger maps in the brain. For example, the hand is capable of extremely intricate and differentiated movements and perceptions. Consequently, the brain devotes a very large area to perceiving and controlling it.

By contrast, the brain doesn't devote as much space to mapping areas with smaller movement or sensation demands, such as the middle of the back or elbow. Just as you would need a very large and detailed map to get around New York City compared to a small town in Iowa, you need a much bigger and detailed map to use your hand than your elbow. Check out the picture on the next page. It's a cross-section of the part of the brain that perceives the body, with body parts drawn in proportion to the size of the maps. Note that all the body parts used for very refined perception, such as the hands and lips, are disproportionately large.

Another indication that good maps are essential for movement and body sense is they grow larger when placed under demand. If you put in enough practice playing a musical instrument, or some other activity that requires extreme precision in the sensation or movements of the fingers, the brain maps for your fingers will grow observably larger.[28] This growth can happen fairly quickly — four days of practice in Braille is enough to reveal (temporary) changes in the brain.[29]

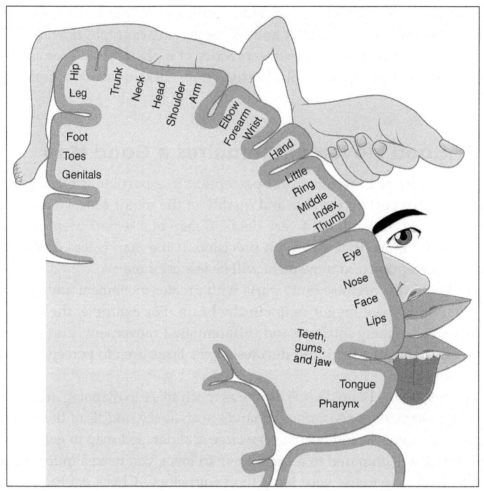

Cross-section of sensory maps, with body parts drawn in proportion to map size.

Maps and imagery

Here's an interesting proof of the significance of the body maps for movement skill. Visualizing performance of a skill will improve performance. It will also cause objective changes in the brain maps that relate to the skill. For example, visualizing piano practice, dart throwing and even lifting weights can increase performance, often to a degree that is comparable to actual practice.[30]

Visualization works because the same maps that execute a movement are also used to imagine it. Therefore, on the neural level, making a movement and thinking about a movement are not so different. Try to imagine writing your name in the air with your dominant hand. Now try with the non-dominant hand. Did it take longer the second time? That's because the skill of imagination lives in the same maps that control the movement.

The connection between movement and thinking about movement mirrors another theme that consistently emerges from the study of the body maps — our ability to control movement is intimately related to our ability to perceive it. As stated by Michael Merzenich, one of the pioneer researchers in the neuroplasticity revolution, "The feelings and the thoughts about movement are inseparable from the movement itself."[31]

Maps are built by movement

The raw information used to build the maps comes from sensation. You can sense the effects of mechanoreception on your maps by doing a simple experiment. Try to imagine the exact position of your left collarbone — where it attaches to the sternum, its shape as it goes over to the shoulder joint. How clear is the picture in your mind's eye?

Now take the fingers of your right hand and trace along the collarbone from the sternum to the shoulder. Feel the top and bottom until you have outlined its shape and contour. Now take your hand away and try again to imagine its position and shape.

You will probably notice it's now easier to perceive the position of the left clavicle compared to the right. That is because as you touched it, you stimulated the mechanoreceptors there. They sent some signals to the parts of the brain that map the clavicle and, for at least a few moments, that map was lit up by a little neural activity. The excitement of the map made it easier for you to perceive the position of the clavicle.[32]

That's only temporary, of course. In order to make long-term changes in your body maps, you need to place demands on them consistently over a period of time. When a certain movement is used repeatedly in a coordinated way, there are actual physical changes in the part of the brain that controls that movement.

Maps are blurred by lack of movement

If the neural maps created for a certain purpose are not getting used, they will eventually get recruited to perform some other function. For example, blind people don't use their visual cortex to process visual data, so it eventually starts getting involved in processing other sensory data from hearing and touch. (This can lead to seemingly superhuman powers like echolocation — the ability to know where things are through making noises and listening for echos.)

Thus, the health of the brain maps follows the same rule as other structures in the body: Use it or lose it. Sensory maps lose their clarity if they are not fed adequate information from the periphery. And the motor maps will get less precise and differentiated if we do not engage in precise differentiated movement.

In a famous study illustrating this principle, researchers sewed together two fingers on a monkey, so they had to work as one unit. After some time passed, microelectrodes revealed that the two fingers were now mapped in the brain as one unit instead of two.[33]

The lesson is that if you don't use a particular movement or perception for a certain period of time, you may effectively forget how to make that movement or perception. This is sometimes called "sensory motor amnesia."

In modern life, there are certain parts of the body that tend to get effectively "sewn together" like the fingers on the monkey. Many people habitually move certain multisegmental areas of their spine as one big block, as opposed to a chain with differentiated movement at each segment. After a while, these areas will be represented in the brain as ... one big block. More sophisticated and precise movement in these areas becomes impossible, because there are no maps to sense and control them. When we mobilize our spines into movements we haven't made for a while, we might imagine that any resulting benefits are related to physically breaking through areas that are "sticky" or adhered together. But a better explanation might be that we are simply reminding the brain of the places it can move.

Pain and the body maps

People with chronic pain have altered cortical maps. They also have relatively poor performance on tasks designed to test perception or movement of the body, such as two-point discrimination tests and voluntary lumbopelvic control.

There are a few common sense reasons why pain would tend to "blur" the motor sensory maps. First, pain discourages movement, which reduces proprioceptive signaling. Second, the presence of nociception (signals indicating tissue damage) will tend to compete with proprioception for the brain's attention. This can lead to "sensory gating," which means that sensory information will get ignored if it is deemed less important than other sensory information.

For example, if your ankle is sprained, you will probably move it less, which means less sensory signaling to the brain about certain joint positions. Further, any proprioceptive signaling will tend to get ignored because the brain is focusing its attention on nociception. Thus, the maps for the ankle may lose clarity, which reduces coordination, which makes it more likely for the ankle to get sprained again. The end result of this vicious cycle is that the brain gets very good at perceiving pain in the ankle, and not so good at perceiving joint position and controlling movement.

Not only can pain cause alterations in the maps, but alterations in the maps can cause pain. The most dramatic example is when people with an amputated limb experience pain in the missing limb. Even though the limb is gone, the virtual limb in the brain lives on, and can be stimulated by cross talk from nearby neural activity.[34] This often results in severe pain. An amazing treatment for phantom limb pain involves placing the remaining limb in a mirror box in a way that fools the brain into thinking the missing limb is alive and well! A great example of how the health of the virtual bodies is just as important as the actual bodies.

Researchers have found they can cause pain by creating unusual sensory illusions using mirrors or other perceptual tricks. On the basis of these and other experiments, many experts believe that "smudges" in the body maps may be a contributing factor in many chronic pain conditions, and that fixing these problems is a potential treatment. We will discuss this in more detail in the chapter on pain.

Now that we've discussed why we want accurate maps for movement and perception, let's look at how we can change them for the better.

Why Do the Maps Change?

The nervous system is constantly changing and adapting throughout its lifespan to learn and improve function. But even though the brain is designed to be responsive to its environment, it is not molded by each new input like a piece of clay. Of course, it can resist changes in its organization that are undesirable.

For a given person, the current organization of their sensory motor maps *already* reflects a lifetime of effort to organize them in an optimal way to perform functional goals. We would not expect further change without good reason. Let's look at the factors that would likely cause the sensory motor maps to change.

Repetition, habits and learning

We know from common experience that repetition is a key factor in learning, skill acquisition, memory and habit formation. If the brain is repeatedly placed under demand to perform a certain function, including interpreting sensory information or executing a movement, it will reorganize to improve performance. There are some very simplified rules of neuroplasticity that help explain what is happening on the neural level as the brain reorganizes in response to repetitive stimuli.

The ability of one neuron to excite another depends on the strength of their synaptic connection. Repeated use of a connection will strengthen it. The complex physiology that governs the strength of neural connections is sometimes simplified into the following rule: "Neurons that fire together, wire together." (This process and similar processes are also called long-term potentiation and hebbian plasticity.)

This rule means the more we engage in a certain pattern of neural activity, the more facilitated that pattern will become. Neuroscientists believe this process is fundamental to learning, memory and habit formation.

The facilitation of a neural pathway that results from repetition can be likened to carving a groove through snow while skiing down a mountain. On the first pass, all pathways down the mountain are equally likely. But on the second pass, you are more likely to fall into the groove created on the first pass. The more times the same path is traveled, the deeper the groove becomes and the easier it is to follow that same pathway.[35]

In the context of movement, this means the more times we use a certain pattern of brain activity to control a movement, the more automatic that pattern of movement becomes, and the less stimulus is required to trigger it.

Movement habits

Movement automaticity has advantages and disadvantages. On the plus side, the pattern can be invoked and maintained with a minimum of effort and conscious attention. It is very useful for a tennis player to be able to automatically execute the same stroke every time without consciously controlling each aspect of the movement.

On the negative side, if that same tennis player wanted to change his or her technique to prevent pain or improve performance, the automaticity of the movement makes change more difficult. The problem now is not just to build new grooves, but to inhibit old ones. This is why many coaches make a point of ensuring their students are using proper technique *before* it is repeated enough times to become habitual and more difficult to change. To use the skiing down the mountain analogy, they ensure that students are taking the right path down before it becomes deeply grooved.

These same rules about repetition and habit also apply to perception. The more times the brain interprets a particular bit of sensory information in a particular way, the more likely it is to arrive at that same interpretation in the future. The perception becomes more automatic and efficient, so the brain recognizes the meaning of the information quicker and with less effort.

Again this has advantages and disadvantages. A skilled dancer can anticipate the movements of her partner after half a step because she has seen what follows that half step thousands of times. An elite quarterback can read the whole field with a brief glance. The more skilled we become in interpreting the meaning of sensory information, the fewer pixels we need to fill out the remainder of a very detailed and useful picture.

But the same shortcuts and automaticity that allows us to form quick perceptions can also lead us astray. By guessing at patterns before they are fully supported by sensory data, we can be deceived. Magicians exploit our habits and perceptual shortcuts to make us see things that aren't even there.

Similarly, as we will discuss more in the pain section, we can develop habits in the way we perceive threat to the body, so pain can arise in the absence of any real danger.

Change is a two-stage process

The neural grooves or facilitated patterns of brain activity that underlie memory and habit are formed in what prominent neuroplasticity researcher Alvaro Pascual-Leon describes as a two-stage process.[36]

In the first stage, as a new skill is being learned, the brain uses *existing* neural connections and strengthens them to create the desired patterns of brain activity. This leads to a temporary facilitation of these pathways and a moderate increase in skill.

In the second stage, *new* neural connections are created through dendritic sprouting and arborization. This process requires more time, energy and practice, but results in greater and longer lasting changes in function. The skills can be executed quicker, more efficiently, and with less conscious attention.[37] Further, the new maps are effectively permanent. The increased efficiency and permanence of the skill is in part due to the fact that the brain has created a custom neural map for its execution.[38] The new map moves away from the higher brain regions involved in focused attention and decision-making to the subcortical regions. It also changes from involving broadly distributed brain activity to more focused activity.[39]

The two-stage process concept is consistent with conventional motor learning theory, which observes that skill development proceeds in stages. First, in what is called the cognitive stage, performance of the skill requires great mental effort and conscious attention. After enough practice, performance of the skill eventually becomes "automatic," and requires almost no conscious attention or effort at all.

This two-stage pattern is also easily recognized from common experience. For example, when we cram for a test, we can quickly accumulate great amounts of knowledge sufficient to pass the test, but the information will soon be forgotten. The knowledge was encoded in neural structures developed for some other purpose, and the strength of their connections quickly fades. The maps were only temporary.

On the other hand, any skill we develop to the expert level, such as fluency in a language or mastery of an instrument, will always be there to some extent. Even after years of neglect, the foundation will remain, and the prior level of skill can be recovered fairly easily with just a little brushing up. The maps are fairly permanent.

If we want to understand how to make improvements in the brain activity that controls how we move and feel, it is useful to keep the concepts of grooves, habits and stages of learning in mind. This can help us imagine what kinds of neural adaptations and what levels of practice are necessary to accomplish different types of movement goals.

For example, it is obvious that if we want to learn a new sport from scratch we will need to build totally new maps to perform the skill at a high level, and this can be expected to take quite a bit of time and effort. On the other hand, if we just need to brush up on some rusty skills that are already supported by long-term maps, we can expect quick progress. Other movement goals might require us to get *out* of a bad habit that has previously been established, and this might be one of the hardest tasks to achieve.

Based on these ideas, we might distinguish four different kinds of movement goals that associate with four different kinds of map alteration. They are:

1. Maintaining a groove

2. Finding a lost groove

3. Building a new groove

4. Getting out of a bad groove

These constructs are obviously rather speculative and metaphorical, but I think they are a useful way to simplify some concepts that would otherwise be too complex to understand. Here is some more detail on these four categories.

1. Maintaining a groove: map activation

The quickest (and most temporary) way to affect the sensory motor maps is to excite them. Recall the exercise earlier in this chapter which involved touching the collarbone, thereby exciting its sensory maps, and temporarily experiencing an increased ability to accurately perceive its location in space.

This type of temporary excitement is an important part of warming up for a skilled activity. Many coaches make "activation" drills part of their warm-up. These are often designed to increase recruitment of certain muscles (e.g.

the glutes) that are believed to be prone to inhibition. Part of what is getting "activated" here are the neural maps that govern movements. In terms of the groove analogy, these exercises will not create a *new* groove, but will help you get into the *right* groove for what you want to do.

In the context of everyday life, these brief activations also help maintain the integrity of the maps, which, just like the body, operate on a use it or lose it basis. If you want to preserve your current ability to squat, reach overhead, extend the chest, and rotate the spine, you need to use these movement patterns at some minimum frequency to prevent them from getting rusty. Prevention is always easier than cure, so this will only involve a minor amount of work. For most people, a couple minutes every day or two is probably sufficient.

2. Finding a lost groove: repairing old maps

Imagine returning to an activity at which you were formerly expert. For example, speaking a language, playing an instrument, or competing in a sport for the first time in years. Your skills will be rusty, but you will make very quick progress with a little practice. You can think of this as clearing away some overgrowth on the well-worn neural pathways you established many years ago.

Finding a lost groove might occur in the context of rehabbing movement after an injury. Imagine a healthy and athletic person who has sprained an ankle and has now developed back pain. Perhaps the limping caused some compensatory protective movements or stiffness in the back that are now aggravating it.

Maybe this person just needs to revisit the well-established sensory motor patterns that he used successfully for years, but then put on hold for a month or two while the ankle healed. He might be helped by any form of exercise that encourages him to retrieve those old motor patterns — yoga, Pilates, running, mobility drills. Like a computer problem that can be fixed by just rebooting, there are a wide variety of solutions that can help.

This quick recovery of proper movement patterns is an example of what Gray Cook might call a "reset," or what Thomas Hanna would call curing "sensory motor amnesia." It accounts for the easy and quick successes in improving movement that we see from a variety of interventions.

3. Carving a new groove

When you learn something new, you cannot perform it with automaticity and efficiency until you complete the time-consuming process of building new maps. Learning to speak a new language, develop new sports skills, or play the violin takes time.

In the therapeutic context, we are not usually trying to learn *new* movements, but to recover the previous quality of old movements, like squatting, breathing, reaching, or running. These are all movements that were presumably working just fine at some earlier time in our life, and therefore we must have built some quality maps for them. So why can't they always be recovered just as easily as a neglected language or instrument skill?

One answer is that the structure of the body changed in some way during the time of neglect. If an ankle won't fully dorsiflex due to disuse or injury, then the old squat pattern that relied on full dorsiflexion isn't so useful anymore, no matter how intelligently the muscles are used to execute the movement.

Or consider someone who has not thrown a baseball for twenty years. In the meantime, her shoulder has probably gone through many changes — less muscle, degeneration in the bones, or partial tears in the rotator cuff. The maps for safe and effective throwing can be accessed, but they were built to perceive and control a much younger shoulder! The maps may need to go through some substantial adjustment to accommodate the new structure. As they say, the brain remembers but the body forgets. A new groove for throwing must be created to suit the new shoulder. This takes more time than just brushing up on an old skill.

The situation would probably be different if she had continued to throw at least a little bit over the years. The gradual changes in the structure of the shoulder would have been accommodated by gradual changes in the brain maps that perceive and control it.

In general, it is probably safe to say that the longer a certain movement pattern has been neglected over time, and the more structural changes that have occurred in the interim period, the more work there is to be done to adjust and optimize the maps that perceive and control the movement. On the other hand, if we stay active, the brain will continually make the minor updates necessary to account for any ongoing changes in structure.

4. Getting out of a bad groove

We all know it is hard to change a bad habit. Many of our greatest struggles in life involve trying to break addictions, compulsions, or deeply ingrained behaviors. Unlearning can be more difficult than learning, because the challenge is to inhibit connections that have already grown strong in the brain. What do the basic concepts of neuroplasticity tell us about how we can change a bad habit of movement or perception?

There is a corollary to the rule about neurons firing together and wiring together: Neurons that "fire apart, wire apart." This rule gives insight into how a habit can be broken.

Imagine that every time you reach for a computer mouse you also tense your neck. Soon the maps that control these separate movements will develop an intimate connection. Just like Pavlov's dogs salivated each time the dinner bell rang, your neck will tense every time you reach for a mouse. Even worse, if you experience a little bit of pain each time, the neural maps for the pain will start to strengthen their connection to the maps for reaching. The result is that reaching for the mouse is so closely connected with neck tension and pain that performing one necessarily invokes the others.

Moshe Feldenkrais would refer to the tensing of the neck as a "parasitic movement." It is like a reflex — there is no ability to inhibit it, and perhaps no awareness it is even occurring. (By the way, not all parasitic movements are a problem. Michael Jordan stuck out his tongue every time he shot a basketball, but the ball still went into the hoop often enough.)

At the neural level, the way we inhibit the undesirable connection between the parasite map and its host is to activate one while keeping the other quiet. This will cause the maps to fire apart, and therefore wire apart. To use the Pavlov example, this means we would just need to ring the dinner bell without serving dinner. After enough rings without dinner, the association starts to break, and the dogs stop salivating upon hearing the bell.

To inhibit the parasitic connection between mouse reaching and neck tensing, we would need to engage in as many reps as possible of one without the other. This might require moving very slowly and carefully with a good degree of conscious attention and control. After enough reps, the parasitic connection will be weakened. (But old habits die hard!)

This rule works for perception as well. If your brain has developed a very strong association between turning your head to the left and experiencing pain, you can start to break that connection by finding any way possible to turn your head to look to the left without pain. This might involve using your hands to turn the head, or turning the shoulders around the head instead of the head around the shoulders, or rolling the head on the floor in a different relationship to gravity. To the extent that any of these methods allow head turning without pain, they will serve to break neural connections between the movement and the perception of threat. Many of the lessons at the end of this book use this strategy.

The key role of attention

Attention is an important factor in neuroplasticity, because it strongly affects what types of information from the body are likely to cause changes in the brain.

The brain is constantly bombarded with information about the position and movement of the body, and it does not have the power to fully process all of it. Fortunately, most of it is redundant or irrelevant to the performance of functional goals. Therefore, the brain filters out most sensory information, and processes only the bits it needs to form the perceptions it considers useful.

One example of such filtering is the phenomenon of inattentional blindness, which describes the failure to see conspicuous objects in the field of vision. One famous study asked people to watch a video of a basketball game and count the number of passes. Because they were focusing their attention on this task, almost half the participants failed to notice a man in a gorilla suit run right into the middle of the TV screen. Not surprisingly, they were completely amazed to see the gorilla on replay, and could not believe they had missed it in the first place.[40] Magicians are experts at using inattentional blindness to prevent their audience from seeing how their tricks are done, which is often quite obvious when attention is directed in the right location. A tragic consequence of inattentional blindness is a car accident that results from talking on a cell phone.

These examples show that direction of attention will dramatically affect which items of sensory data get filtered out, and which become the basis for conscious perceptions.[41] Because attention is a limited resource, we can only perceive a small percentage of what is there to be perceived at a particular moment.

Most of us have experienced the cocktail party effect, whereby we can tune in and out of different conversations at a party based on where we direct our attention. As soon as we start listening in on one conversation, we lose our ability to understand another one.

We can also tune in and out of the different streams of sensory information that are continually arising from all the different parts of the body. Very few of these sensory signals will result in any actual awareness, but you can create awareness in any locality by focusing your attention there.

For example, right now you can focus on:

* The sensation of air passing over your nostrils as you breathe

* The contact of your left sit bone with a chair

* The feeling of your shirt touching your back

Sensory information that was previously being ignored is now processed.[42] This excites neural activity in the parts of the brain responsible for perceiving these areas. And so you perceive things that were previously missed.

This is why focused attention is one of the key requirements for practice that maximizes neuroplasticity and associated motor learning. The type of deep practice or flow state that produces the greatest gains in skill is characterized by tunnel vision on the activity at hand.[43] World-class performers have an exceptional ability to spend a great deal of time in this state. People who are less skilled at focusing their attention will learn more slowly. Interestingly, some performance experts argue that what appears to be inborn natural talent at a particular activity is actually better described as a natural ability to engage in deep practice.

As we will discuss later in the book, the ability to focus attention and filter information with attention is trainable, as shown by studies on meditation. And there are many traditional forms of movement practice such as tai chi, yoga and martial arts which use focused attention on sensory feedback from movement as a means to improve the health of the mind and the body. The exercises recommended at the end of this book utilize the direction of attention as a primary component.

Direction of attention

The direction in which attention is focused is also relevant to motor learning. There is a substantial body of research indicating that in a wide variety of circumstances, an *external* focus of attention leads to faster motor learning than an *internal* focus of attention.[44]

What is the difference? An internal focus means the student thinks about the movement of his body during execution of a task. An external focus means the student places attention on the effects of his movement in the environment.

For example, during a vertical jump, you could think about extending your hips and knees (internal focus), or you could think about pushing your feet into the floor (external). To do an abdominal curl up, you could think about flexing and shortening the abs, or raising the head to see the feet. When throwing a dart, you could think about flexion at the wrist, or simply focus attention on hitting the target.

Most of the research comparing external to internal focus finds that external promotes faster motor learning. However, there is some research and expert opinion indicating that novices might, in some circumstances, benefit more from internal cueing.[45] The logic of shifting attention externally once skills are more automatic is consistent with the concept of the stages of motor learning, where motor control initially requires significant conscious attention and then proceeds to a more automatic stage of execution.

My interpretation is that external cues evoke motor patterns that are already well learned, and that internal cues encourage the use of motor patterns that are novel. Thus, although external cues should probably be preferred in most instances, internal cues might be useful for getting out of bad movement habits or for building new ones.

Therefore, whether you choose to use an external or internal focus of attention during movement will depend on whether you are trying to perfect a motor program that is already well developed, trying to learn a new pattern, or trying to break an old pattern. As a general rule, external would be preferred in the context of performance, and internal might have more application in the context of rehab.

One way or the other, attention is a tool that will have different effects depending on where it is directed. The best approach is to experiment with different places to focus attention and compare results.

Novel distractions

Novel sensory input gets the brain's attention.[46] Most of the proprioceptive information coming from the body is redundant to other sensory information, including information that was reported from the same area only a few seconds ago. But a change in the flow of information indicates something interesting.

Imagine sitting in your chair for an hour. The receptors in the skin of your back are constantly firing and telling your brain they are in contact with the back of the chair. After a second or two, this information is completely redundant and will likely get ignored. Your brain will only become interested when there is a *change*. Imagine a bug crawls across your back. The novelty of the new sensory signaling would get the brain's attention. The result is a very clear perception of the situation, and probably some quick corrective movements. But the bug has not really changed the *volume* of sensory information coming from the back — what has changed is the *meaning* the brain assigns to the sensory information.

This suggests that novel movements will get the brain's attention and excite the body maps more than familiar movements. It is interesting to note that almost any intervention intended to treat pain and improve quality of movement involves novel stimulus. Ultrasound, massage, manipulation, kinesiotape, instrument assisted soft tissue manipulation, foam rolling, joint mobility drills, yoga poses, stretching, acupuncture, and corrective exercise all involve movements, postures or touch that is unfamiliar.

Functional relevance

Although novel information will catch the brain's attention for an instant or two, we would not expect it to cause long term changes in the maps unless it serves to improve a function. For example, ultrasound may feel interesting to the brain for awhile, and may lead to changes in the way the stimulated area moves and feels. But the changes are likely to be short term if the novel information is not relevant to the performance of some functional task. Once the brain determines the new inputs are just a curiosity as opposed to some key data that helps solve a movement puzzle, it will stop using that information as a way to reorganize the motor sensory maps.

This is why passive massage treatments often have temporary effects that diminish as the stimulus becomes more familiar and loses its novelty.[47] Like a meaningless relationship, the treatment soon loses its magic, and new novel distractions are sought. Chiropractor and movement coach Dr. Eric Cobb calls this the "parking lot effect." Clients feel great as they leave the office after an adjustment, but are already stiffening up by the time they reach their car.

The situation is different with active movement based therapies that help the brain create better function.[48] They can be the start of a process to create long term change in the way the brain perceives and moves a particular area.

Recall the amazing feeling of performing some physical challenge correctly for the first time — learning to ride a bike, striking a golf ball in the center, making a proper turn on the ski slope. The sensory experience of the movement makes a very strong impression not because it is *novel*, but because it is associated with a major step forward in function. It's an "aha" moment because the brain immediately recognizes the usefulness of the movement. The associated sensory feedback can now be used as a reference of correctness to judge the accuracy of future movements. The takeaway is that sensory input that is associated with function is far more likely to enable neuroplasticity than sensory input that is merely novel and interesting.

The rule of functional salience has been demonstrated in research examining the use of sensory discrimination training as a means to reduce pain in patients with chronic regional pain syndrome. CRPS patients have disturbed sensory maps and a reduced ability to discriminate between two different types of tactile stimuli. For example, it is harder for them to tell the difference between a pen cap and a wine cork.

One study found that tactile discrimination training created significant reductions in pain and disability in CRPS patients. *But touch stimulation alone created no effect in the control group.* So both groups received the same amount of novel sensory input, but only the patients who considered that information relevant to improvement of a particular function were able to change their maps and derive benefit.[49]

In the context of doing some form of movement exercise to improve coordination, we can speculate that it will be more effective if it can be tied to some function the brain considers useful.[50] Many passive techniques like massage or foam rolling might be very interesting to the brain for a while, but they do not suggest solutions to movement problems. By contrast, squatting in a different way might be both novel AND part of a solution to a movement challenge that arises every day.

Feedback

Improvement of motor control and associated changes to the motor maps requires feedback about whether a particular movement was successful in accomplishing its intended goal. If I want to improve my free throw shooting in basketball, I need to know if the ball goes in the hoop.

The nervous system is always receiving sensory feedback about the results of motor commands. The feedback can be compared to the *predicted* feedback in order to assess if the movement was successful and learn from mistakes.[51] So every movement is an experiment — there is a hypothesis, data is gathered, and there is an analysis of whether the movement was successful. This is how we learn.

In many endeavors it is very easy to obtain immediate and useful feedback about the success of a certain movement, and in these tasks it is relatively easy to improve skill with mere repetition. When we swing at a baseball, we know immediately if the ball was struck. When we pluck the string of a guitar, we know if it sounds right. The immediacy and obviousness of the feedback in each of these tasks means that practice will create quick improvement, even when the quality of practice is poor.

But there are other classes of movement that do not create feedback that is immediate, obvious and objective, and in these cases it is harder to make improvements. *Unfortunately, these are exactly the types of movements that are often relevant in a therapeutic context.*

For example, consider the movement or postural goals that are frequently the subject of physical therapy or corrective exercise. We may try to change :

* Breathing patterns

* Posture

* Gait

* Muscle activation patterns used for stability

* Proper centration or alignment of the joints during movement

* The distribution of work between joints to create multisegmental ranges of motion

In each case, the relative "correctness" of the posture or movement at issue does not result in some objective manifestation that is easily visible in the external world. Whether posture is good or bad, breathing is shallow or deep, or an overhead reach uses more serratus anterior or levator scapula, there are no obvious effects in the environment that reveal whether the movement was done "wrong" or "right." We don't see whether the ball goes in the hoop.

In the absence of a coach to provide feedback, improving these movements will be more difficult. One solution is to impose some constraint on movement that will make the difference between right and wrong more obvious. For example, if you wanted to encourage more thoracic extension and less cervical extension when looking up, placing the hands behind the head will encourage the desired pattern. This strategy of using constraints is used in the lessons at the end of this book, and is discussed in more detail in the chapter on developmental movements.

Another approach is to pay closer attention to sensory feedback from the body, to make it easier to discern subtle differences in the comfort level or efficiency of doing a movement. For example, we might not notice that our breathing is shallow or effortful if our attention is focused elsewhere, but spending a few minutes paying careful attention to the differences between alternate ways of breathing might increase awareness. Maybe one method is slightly more relaxing, takes less effort, or avoids a minor discomfort in the neck with each inhalation. These are all subtle differences that could easily be missed without the focus of specific attention.

If a preferred method is found, either through self-exploration or specific direction from a coach, the sensory feedback associated with that method can be used as a reference for correctness for future breathing. It forms the new standard by which breathing is judged, which alerts the nervous system to the presence of errors that need correction. Of course, this process needs to occur on an unconscious level to be effective and sustainable.

The lessons in this book are a way to learn preferable ways to move *without* the presence of a coach giving constant feedback. Part of the intent is to encourage exploration of different movements, focus of attention on subtle differences between the movements, and repetition of movements that feel best. The hopeful result is increased skill in using internal feedback as a way to improve comfort and performance.

Exercise, reward and motivation

Although this book has a "brain-based" perspective, and focuses on "top down" methods of optimizing movement, it must be acknowledged that the brain and the body work together, and that one affects the other. In fact, one of the biggest factors that facilitates neuroplasticity is exercise. Even if it's mindless!

Numerous lines of research show that exercise, in particular aerobic exercise, causes the release of chemicals in the brain that assist growth of new neural pathways.[52] Thus, studies have shown that various forms of learning and memorization are improved after a bout of exercise.

The presence of reward seems to have a similar effect. The brain's reward system makes us feel good when we engage in activities deemed to be useful for survival and procreation. This is why food, exercise, sex and social bonding feel inherently good. Not surprisingly, we learn faster when we feel rewarded during the learning process. Like exercise, the chemicals released during the experience of reward facilitate neuroplasticity. This is one of the reasons why engaging in play can speed learning. (Play will be discussed more in the chapter on development.)

Summary

Let's see if we can boil down the information in this chapter into some big takeaways. Following is brief summary of the major points.

* Perception and movement are controlled in part through the motor sensory maps in the brain, which are patterns of neural activity that often occur in discrete areas.

* The cortical maps that govern perception and motor control are closely connected and mutually dependent. Therefore, the act of perceiving the body is dynamically linked with controlling it and vice versa.

* The structure and function of the motor sensory maps are constantly adapting over our lifetime to optimize the performance of functional goals. This process of adaptation is called neuroplasticity.

* One basic principle of neuroplasticity is that neurons that fire together wire together and neurons that fire apart wire apart. This means that if two maps are always used simultaneously, they will develop connections. If they are used separately, the connections weaken. This is part of how we learn and form habits. And break habits.

* Neuroplasticity happens in a two-stage process. In the first stage, which is more temporary, existing neural connections are "unmasked" and strengthened to create the desired pattern of neural activity. Moving through this stage requires conscious attention.

* In the second stage, new neural connections are created that are more permanent. Building the new connections requires effort and

repetition, but will eventually result in performance that requires little to no conscious attention.

* The increased automaticity and efficiency of deeply grooved motor sensory maps have advantages and disadvantages. They make the execution of certain movements or perceptions more quick, efficient and automatic. However, they can also create habits that effectively prevent the use of alternative movement and perception options.

* Maintaining existing maps is quick and easy. They only need to be occasionally activated with the appropriate activity.

* Updating maps or brushing up on old skills requires more work than maintenance, but is easier than building new maps from scratch.

* Many of the movements we are trying to recover with physical therapy or corrective exercise were at some point in our lives deeply ingrained. The amount of work required to recover them will depend on how long they have been neglected and how much the structure of the body has changed in the interim.

* The greatest challenge in improving movement or perception is in breaking habits that are deeply ingrained. This might require very slow and progressive work.

* Focus of attention has a strong effect on which sensory information the nervous system will process and interpret as opposed to filter and ignore. Thus, focus of attention on the sensory information resulting from movement is an important way to modulate perception and motor control related to that movement.

* Novel movements and sensations are more likely to receive attention than movements or sensations that are redundant or familiar.

* Sensory information that is relevant to the accomplishment of functional goals is more likely to result in learning.

* We learn to move better by conducting movement experiments, where sensory feedback is compared to predictions about movement consequences. Thus, receiving immediate, objective and accurate feedback about the results of the movement is critical to motor learning.

* In some circumstances, feedback about the correctness of a particular movement or perception is easily obtained, because it is obvious in the external world. Improvement in these activities will occur naturally with repetition even in the absence of deep quality practice.

* Other movements, including many activities of everyday life like posture or breathing, do not provide obvious external and objective feedback about the correctness of the movement. In the absence of coaching, improvement of these activities is more difficult and will not necessarily result from repetition. The feedback that is necessary for improvement requires exercises that we impose appropriate constraints and augment feedback, and a heightened degree of awareness in regard to sensory information indicating effort, comfort and efficiency.

* Exercise, reward and motivation facilitate learning.

We will discuss how to use these ideas to develop practical movement strategies in Chapter 7!

CHAPTER 4

MOTOR DEVELOPMENT AND PRIMAL PATTERNS

"No phenomenon can be understood without carefully considering how it emerged."

— Nikolai Bernstein

DURING THE FIRST TWO YEARS of life, babies develop from a quivering blob on the floor, to creatures that can roll over, sit, crawl, squat, walk, manipulate objects and drive their parents crazy. The rate of motor learning is extremely fast and very impressive. Toddlers squat with the perfection of Olympic weightlifters. Their head carriage and posture would please any physical therapist. And their movements have the grace and simplicity of a Zen monk. The amazing thing is these optimal movement patterns emerge without any instruction whatsoever.

This should make us curious about how an infant learns to move so well and so quickly. With that in mind, let's take a look at some aspects of infant motor development that might inform our efforts to improve movement as adults.

Developmental Patterns are Building Blocks

Infants develop movement by progressively learning a series of fundamental movement patterns, which form the building blocks for more complex movements.

For example, while lying on the ground and sitting in various positions, an infant learns to stabilize her head so she can see the world. The motor patterns for head stabilization become a building block for the postural control required in standing and walking.[53] While reaching to grab interesting objects, she learns the arm/trunk coordination patterns that are later used to crawl and walk, and eventually throw and climb.

As she rolls from back to front, one leg provides support while the other moves through space, a skill that forms the basis for locomotion. In crawling, she uses a cross-lateral pattern of limb movement that carries over to walking. And in squatting, she learns patterns of triple extension and flexion that are fundamental to almost any powerful movement in standing.[54]

The fundamental movement patterns learned in infancy are referred to by various names: motor primitives, synergies, primal patterns, and developmental patterns. They can be thought of as neural control programs that can be combined in various ways to generate a large repertoire of movements.[55]

In this sense, movement is like a language. The basic motor patterns are like letters or simple words that can be combined to form more complex sentences. In spoken language, we can communicate an infinite variety of thoughts from relatively few words. Similarly, the complex and varied movements we see in sport and dance can all be broken down into far fewer basic movement patterns — gait, squats, reaches, rotations, etc. An arabesque in dance looks pretty similar to the backswing of a free kick in soccer because they are built from the same basic motor primitives.

This combinatorial system makes the formation of complex structures simpler in terms of neural control.[56] If we had to remember a different word for each thought we could think, our brain would be overwhelmed with the difficulty of storing and retrieving the right word for the right thought. It is far easier to remember a limited amount of words and then combine them. Imagine how much easier it is to remember the phone numbers of seven friends than to remember one forty-nine digit number.

It is the same with movement. It is simpler for the nervous system to rely on a small number of general movement patterns that can be assembled together to form more complex movements.

One implication of this system is when a foundational building block is missing or compromised, the entire structure built on top will suffer. If you are missing some very basic words or letters in your language vocabulary, there are many sentences you will struggle to make. Similarly, if your movement vocabulary is missing one or more important motor primitives, many everyday movements will be compromised.

Thus, if you had the choice of improving one movement, you would choose one that had broad carryover to many other movements, as opposed to one that is highly specialized. For example, if I improve my squat, I will probably also improve my golf swing, my jump shot, and my tennis serve, because these activities are all supported by a basic squat pattern. I will also be more comfortable and functional in my activities of daily living, because I am getting into chairs and picking things off the floor all day. Better squatting could reduce mechanical stress on the hips, knees and low back.

By contrast, if I improve some specific skill, like hitting a tennis serve, I will be better at serving ... but probably nothing else. So if we want to train movement, it is a good idea to train foundational movements, as opposed to highly complex and specialized movements that are specific to only one context. It is therefore no surprise that in corrective exercise, physical therapy, and functional training, it is usually fundamental movements that are emphasized.

What movements are developmental? Some obvious choices would be breathing, head control, reaching, squatting, rolling, crawling, and creeping. If an adult challenges his competence in these movements, he is likely to encourage his brain to retrieve and brush up on some primal movement patterns that may be neglected.

But babies didn't learn these movement patterns by rehearsing or performing them on purpose. The patterns emerged in the context of a *process*. I would argue that it is more useful for adults to re-create that process, as opposed to reenacting some of the movements that emerged out of the process.

There are at least three aspects of the developmental process that would seem useful to an adult:

1. Assuming developmental positions like supine, prone or quadruped.

2. Engaging in developmental tasks like reaching, orienting the head or trying to move from position to position.

3. Moving in a manner that is playful, curious, exploratory, and experimental.

Let's take a look at each of these different aspects of infant motor development in turn.

The Value of Developmental Positions

Primitive movement patterns are learned in developmental positions — supine, prone, quadruped and tripod positions, oblique sitting, kneeling, half-kneeling, squatting, etc. These positions offer several potential advantages to an infant trying to learn useful developmental patterns. And, more importantly, to an adult trying to recover or brush up on such patterns.

Reduction of stability and balance demands

First, developmental postures drastically reduce stability demands compared to standing. On the ground, you have less moving parts, and therefore motor control is simpler. For example, in standing, you need to control the ankles, knees, hips and spine, etc. In a kneeling position, your ankles and feet are taken out of the equation. Further, your center of gravity is lowered closer to your base of support, which increases stability.

As you get even closer to the ground and lie down on your back, stabilization demands are eventually reduced to almost zero. Here, you may find it easier to obtain the full flexion of the hip required for squatting, because your hip muscles are not occupied with bearing weight and creating balance.

Developmental positions also reduce perception of threat related to falling, as well as any related protective mechanisms, such as stiffness, weakness, discomfort and altered coordination. (See Chapter 6 for more on these protective patterns.) Although most of us are not consciously afraid of falling as we walk or squat, there is always some degree of unconscious nervous system activity devoted to preventing a fall. This may involve excess tension and restriction of uncontrolled mobility. To the extent that a developmental position can reduce this protective activity, it can facilitate the recovery of motor patterns that are more difficult to find in standing positions.

Increased proprioceptive input

Another advantage of developmental positions is they increase proprioceptive feedback through contact with the floor. For example, it is easier to perceive the shape and movement of the spinal curves and ribs while lying on the floor than standing in space. On your back, you can sense lumbar flexion by feeling the low back press into the floor. In standing, this form of feedback is not available.

Increased constraints: fewer bad choices

Part of the reason developmental positions improve movement is by *limiting* movement options.[57] Getting on the floor constrains degrees of freedom in a way that *reduces* the number of motor patterns that can be used to perform a particular task. Thus, many potential "bad" patterns of movement are unavailable, while all the "good" ones remain. Developmental patterns are easier to find when they are one of very few potential solutions to a motor challenge.

For example, in crawling, there are fewer choices for how to use the arms than in walking, because one arm must always help support the body weight. Because the hand is fixed to the ground, the arm muscles move the body relative to the arm, instead of the arm relative to the body. The supporting arm will synchronize with the opposite-side supporting leg, so a cross-lateral pattern of limb movement emerges.

In walking, this same cross-lateral pattern *should* be preserved. But because the arms have additional degrees of freedom, it is no longer *required*. The arms don't need to bear weight, so they are free to move out of sync with the opposite side leg. And the muscles on the leading arm are no longer required to "pull" the body forward as in crawling — instead, they can operate to pull the hand back.

To feel how walking can preserve the "closed-chain feel" of the arms in crawling, imagine you are walking with ski poles. The hand that reaches forward, like the crawling arm, to some extent becomes a "fixed point" in space from which the muscles connecting the arm and the trunk can pull the body forward. If you walk this way, you may feel an increased sense of integration of the arms with the trunk during gait.

Thus, walking presents an opportunity to neglect a primal locomotion pattern that is more compulsory in crawling. If this neglect eventually results in some sensory motor amnesia, perhaps crawling can be part of the cure. This is because crawling eliminates the option of using many specific and complex patterns of movement, while preserving only the simple fundamental patterns.

Here's another example. Imagine you are a baby lying flat on your back, and you need to reach to grab an object that is a hanging from a string a few feet in front of your sternum. There are very few combinations of joint movements that will get the job done. Any solution will almost certainly involve:

* Shoulder flexion to ninety degrees

* Scapular protraction

* Rotation of the rib cage to the left

The synergy between shoulder flexion, scapular protraction and thoracic rotation is a very basic reaching pattern that can be used as a building block in many other contexts, including throwing, striking, pushing, running, walking, etc.

Now consider your reaching options in standing, where you have more degrees of freedom. Let's say you are reaching for a glass on a table. You could reach with the primal pattern — shoulder flexion, scapula protraction and thoracic rotation. Or you could avoid all three movements completely. You could reach the glass by bending forward from the waist and flexing the elbow. Or you could turn around and reach backward to get the glass. These patterns get the job done but are very specific and idiosyncratic, useless in all but very limited contexts. The primal pattern is not compulsory.

By contrast, in the supine position, the optimal reaching synergy, which forms a great building block for other movements, is really the only way to get the job done. The tendency for this position to elicit a proper reaching pattern is part of the reason a Turkish get-up is a popular corrective exercise.

We could think of several other examples. While sitting on the ground, if you want a view of what is behind you, you need cooperative and integrated rotation from the neck, scapula, thorax, low back and hips. In standing, you can avoid movement in the thoracic spine and/or the hips by using compensatory movements at the knees, ankles and feet. In prone, if you want to see the world, the thoracic spine needs significant mobility into extension and rotation, and the scapula and neck must coordinate their activity. In standing, you can see above quite easily without much work in the thorax, again by using compensatory motions in the ankles or knees.

In each case, the additional degrees of freedom available in standing make it possible to neglect primal patterns that are more compulsory in developmental positions. The result is the use of an idiosyncratic and specific pattern that might get the job done, but is less efficient, distributes the stress of movement in a non-proportional way, and misses an opportunity to maintain a very important building block for healthy movement. Thus, returning to developmental positions is a way to encourage the use of primal patterns that may be getting ignored in everyday life.

There are some additional factors that beneficially constrain infant movement and which adults *cannot* duplicate by simply returning to developmental positions. An infant has less strength and power relative to an adult, and therefore less capacity to use momentum or ballistic movements to transition between positions. For example, a baby trying to roll from front to back needs to use a very specific motor program to get the job done. An adult can use power to "cheat," avoiding the graceful coordinated movements that are obligatory to the infant.

Thus, it is often useful to create artificial constraints on movement in developmental positions, by requiring that they be accomplished with a minimum of muscular effort and ballistic momentum. One test for the absence of ballistic movement is the ability to reverse the movement in the opposite direction with little or no hesitation. This is why Moshe Feldenkrais considered "reversibility" an important aspect of quality movement.

Resistance is assistance

It is interesting to note that adding resistance to a movement has similar effects to assuming a developmental position, in that it creates constraints on the possible movement patterns that can be used to perform the task. These constraints encourage use of fundamental movement patterns that have broad usefulness, as opposed to specific patterns that are useful only in certain contexts.

For example, if you lift an object from the floor that weighs only a pound, there are literally hundreds of different movements that will get the job done. You could be on tiptoes, reach with an arm behind your back, or bend sideways to pick up the object. The options are endless. Most of them will involve combinations of joint movement that you might never use again.

But if you start adding weight to the object, your range of options narrow, until you are eventually obligated to use a very foundational, powerful and developmental hip hinge/squat pattern. The pattern would not look much different from a toddler picking up a heavy toy.

This is why many trainers who coach the squat have noticed their clients will often *improve* their squat form when weight is added. Trainer Dan John popularized the goblet squat as a way to clean up squat form that looks sloppy when unloaded. The placement of the weight in front of the body is a constraint that prevents the use of poor form. Although the weight is a form of *resistance* to the muscles, it is a form of *assistance* to the nervous system in finding the best movement pattern.

Another constraint that can encourage the use of developmental patterns is the need to move with speed or power. You can jump one inch into the air using a wide variety of movement patterns — off one foot, with the legs crossed, with the hips fully extended as opposed to flexed. But if you want to get your full vertical leap, then you need to assume a classic power-squat position, which would look quite similar to the movement you used to pick up the heavy object. This is why many strength coaches will help a client find the optimal squatting position for their feet by asking them to jump as high as possible.

Locomotion patterns can be beneficially constrained by speeding them up. If you walk slowly, you could walk with your arms and legs moving in a homolateral pattern instead of cross lateral. That is, you could move the left arm forward and back in sync with the left leg instead of the right leg. But as you start to walk faster, the homolateral pattern is almost impossible to maintain, and the cross-lateral pattern will emerge spontaneously. The primal pattern becomes obligatory with speed.

The takeaway message here is that if you continually place yourself in a movement environment with very few constraints — where one movement works just as well as another to accomplish a task, then there is nothing to encourage use of the primal patterns of movement that are the foundation for your function and health. But if you put yourself in situations where use of primal patterns is more obligatory — developmental positions, or movements that require force, speed or power, then you are obligated to maintain and refine these patterns.

Among these different options, returning to developmental positions is one of the easiest and safest ways to create beneficial constraints on movement, because unlike moving with strength, speed and power, it decreases rather than increases perception of threat and the protective mechanism that accompany that perception.

But if you are free of pain, working on movements that create the most speed, power and force — deadlifts, squats, lunges, pushes, pulls, sprints, jumps, throws and kicks — is one way to maintain and even improve good patterns of movement. And you get fit in the process!

The Value of Developmental Tasks

What movements are developmental? As noted before, some obvious choices would be breathing, head control, reaching, squatting, rolling, crawling, creeping, and object manipulation.

Another perspective on developmental movement comes from simply thinking about the goals infants are trying to accomplish, and from what positions. Infants are fairly simple creatures and are usually only interested in doing two basic things — seeing things and grabbing things. They want to get a good view of the world — orient their eyes and ears toward interesting faces, objects and noises. And they want to be able to grasp interesting objects, manipulate them with their hands, and put them in their mouth. And they want to move themselves around to see more interesting things and put more interesting objects in their mouth. That's about it for their functional movement goals!

With that in mind, it is very interesting to note how many developmental movements emerge out of a simple intention to accomplish one or both of these two basic goals from a developmental position. Head control arises out of trying to orient the head toward mommy while on the stomach and in other positions. Rolling can easily arise from a simple intention to see and reach. Squatting patterns are evoked by an intention to put the feet in the mouth while on the back.

Here's an interesting exercise to illustrate. Get into any developmental position and then start trying to reach or see as many things as a baby would be able to reach or see from that position. (No cheating by using more power and strength than is available to a baby.) You will find yourself spontaneously engaging in many developmental movements even without any conscious intention to do so.

* From the prone position, if you start trying to see what is behind you, using only your arms for support, you may find your legs moving into lizard-like creeping movements.

* While lying on your back, reaching for an object on the floor may cause you to roll.

* In sitting, if you slide your hand forward on the floor far enough to reach an object, you may find yourself transitioning to quadruped.

* While in quadruped, looking up, down, right and left will mobilize the entire spine and pelvis into coordinated global patterns of flexion, extension, side flexion and rotation.

* In quadruped, reaching a hand forward to grab an object will encourage a transition into crawling.

* In a bear-crawling position on hands and feet, looking up to see what is in front of you will tend to move you into a squat. Reaching with one hand into as many different parts of the floor or space will be a huge test of balance and integrated coordination in the squat position.

The interesting thing about this exercise is the transitional movements produced by the mere intention to reach or get a view of something are often smoother, more integrated, and more coordinated than the same movements would be if we intended to perform them on purpose. This highlights the fact that babies do not learn movement by trying to learn movement. They learn movement by trying to perform functional tasks, and the movements emerge out of that process. Thus, movement patterns develop not by a top-down process of dictating exactly how they will happen, but by a bottoms-up organic evolutionary process. And central to that process is play.

Play

Children don't learn fundamental movement patterns through work or instruction. Instead, they learn them through play, exploration and experimentation.

Play is commonly defined as an activity that is fun, voluntary, improvisational, absorbing, and without obvious purpose.[58] It can also be understood as the opposite of boring work — something that is done with a specific outcome in mind, under the stress of need, and that takes willpower to continue.

In the natural world, play is an essential part of any significant learning process. All intelligent animals play. The more intelligent the animal, the more it plays. Chimps, dolphins, and dogs play more than snakes, turtles and bugs. Humans are the smartest animals and play the most.

Animals engage in the most play when their educational demands are highest. For example, when it's time to learn the physical skills necessary for hunting, or the social skills required for mating and group membership — these are the exact times when the animal naturally engages in the most play. When an intelligent animal is deprived of play, it will not develop into a normal adult, and will instead experience severe problems with learning and social behavior.

Based on these facts, it is obvious that play is integral to learning, and that play is the best solution to difficult educational problems that evolution has found. In this sense, play presents a bit of a paradox. Why is it so effective in achieving educational outcomes, when its very nature is to ignore the outcome and focus on the process? How does it help us arrive at a destination quickly when it encourages detours? Why does play foster learning? Here are some potential answers.

Neuroplasticity and play

Play involves focused attention, it is rewarding, and it promotes the development of novel movement and perceptions. These are all important preconditions for neuroplasticity. Play also activates brain-derived neurotrophic factor, which stimulates nerve growth.[59] Play seems to have a more widespread effect on the brain than work. Rats who are forced to work at finding their way through a maze experience neural growth in the one specific area of the brain responsible for this task. By contrast, rats placed in an enhanced play environment experience global brain benefits — they have thicker cortexes.[60]

Play helps you move outside the box

Some researchers believe that mammals evolved a motivation to play because it introduces an element of randomness or creativity into problem solving.[61] Because play values variation and novelty as an end in itself, engaging in play is a way to ensure you are always experimenting with new options and thinking outside the box.

In the context of movement, play can be thought of as a safeguard against habitually using the same movement pattern to solve a particular motor challenge and ignoring potentially better solutions.

To use the skiing down the mountain analogy, a very workmanlike or goal oriented mindset would encourage use of the most well grooved path. A more playful process would encourage exploration of alternative pathways, some of which might be faster (once they are practiced a few times).

Thus, we can look at our motivation to play as a natural incentive to experiment with new solutions, even if they don't appear superior at first glance. We could also look at play as a way to "return to the drawing board" or start over from scratch on a movement problem without preconceived notions about the right or wrong way to move.

Play develops resourcefulness and adaptability

Researchers have also noted that playful behavior exposes us to a wide variety of novel circumstances in a way that may teach adaptability and resourcefulness.[62]

Again, to use the skiing down the mountain analogy, someone who is motivated to explore the whole mountain will expose themselves to a wide variety of pathways and terrains. This will promote a creativity and responsiveness that is useful in the real world, which always involves novel challenges.

Michael Merzenich believes one of the major practical takeaways from his pioneering research into neuroplasticity is that "stereotypy is the enemy" and that the brain is best exercised with a variety of movements and challenges. For example, it is preferable to "move to a point in space in 100 different speeds in 100 different ways ... than to move 200 times in the same way to get to that point in space."[63]

Thus, in Merzenich's view, proper movement training would not involve simply repeating the same motion over and over again in the same way. Exploration and variety are more important for real world value, because what the brain really wants is to be able to solve a task in a wide variety of circumstances.

Consider these ideas in the context of training the ability to lower your center of gravity to the ground. If you watch kids move from the floor to standing, you will see them select a different pathway almost every time. But if you watch adults train this movement in a gym, you will see one or maybe two ways to lower the center of gravity — a squat and a lunge. This is the stereotyped movement that Merzenich says is indicative of reduced capacity. Thus, one of the lessons from the science of play is that squatting in the exact same way each time you go to the gym is probably not the best way to optimize your squatting, or anything else.

Louie Simmons is one of the most successful powerlifting coaches in the world. This is a sport that requires only three simple movements in competition: squat, deadlift and bench press. Despite the very small movement vocabulary used on game day, Simmons trains his athletes with constant variety in the way they perform these movements. His rationale: "As soon as your body thinks it has all the answers, you need to start asking different questions."

Although there is very clearly a role for repetitive and sometimes boring drills in getting better at a specific skill, all elite movers attain their status not just through boring drudgery, but through playful creativity, exploration and variation.

✳ Summary

The developmental movement patterns learned in infancy are the building blocks for more complex movements. A modern sedentary life eliminates many of the constraints that require the use of these movements. Thus, there is significant opportunity to neglect them. A primary focus of any program for maintaining or reclaiming movement health should be to ensure that fundamental movement patterns are healthy.

For many people, significant time spent walking, squatting and sitting on the floor will be sufficient to keep these patterns intact. Unfortunately, modern life seems to involve less and less of these activities.

The easiest and safest way to improve or maintain fundamental movement patterns is to recreate the process from which they emerged. A simple three-step template could generate a thousand useful developmental movement lessons.

1. Get into a developmental position such as supine, prone, sidelying, side sitting, long sitting, sitting with the soles of the feet together, kneeling, half kneeling, tall kneeling, quadruped, tripod, or squatting.

2. Engage in some developmental task such as orienting the head to see, reaching for something, or transitioning to a different position.

3. Do the movements in a playful, exploratory manner, with a minimum of muscular effort and momentum, preserving the ability to reverse the movement in the opposite direction. The lessons in Chapter 7 are specific applications of this general strategy.

Activities outside developmental positions can also train fundamental movement patterns, particularly if they involve movements that require strength, speed and power, like running, jumping, climbing, throwing and lifting. Lifting is particularly beneficial if it involves full range of motion compound movements like squats, deadlifts, lunges, pushups, pullups and rows. However, because each of these activities brings the threat of injury, they are more likely to invite protective compensations. (See Chapter 6 for more detail.) In this event, "regressing" to the floor is a good option, with eventual progression to standing being a good goal.

PART II

THE SCIENCE OF FEELING BETTER

CHAPTER 5

THE SCIENCE OF PAIN

"Pain is an opinion."
— Vilayanur Ramachandran

A WOMAN GOES TO HER DOCTOR in terrible back pain. It came on for no obvious reason. Her doctor arranges for an MRI that reveals a herniated disc. She doesn't want surgery, so she goes to a physical therapist, who says her core is weak and she needs to do core strengthening exercises. The exercises don't help, so she sees a chiropractor, who says her spine needs to be realigned by adjustments. This works for a few days, and then seems to make things worse.

A friend tells her to see a reflexologist. She is skeptical, but after the reflexologist presses certain points on her foot, her back pain disappears. She is ecstatic but the pain returns two weeks later and soon moves to a different part of her back. Months pass and she continues to seek new solutions — acupuncture, yoga, massage and stretching. Each provider offers a different explanation for her pain and a different treatment. The treatments address alleged problems with fascia, chi, toxins, trigger points, strength, flexibility and motor control. Her pain rises and falls, moves from place to place, but remains a problem.

She becomes very frustrated that no one is able to give her a clear explanation for her problem and how to treat it. She has no idea what to think, no way to explain her symptoms, and no way to guess what might help her feel better in the future. She is confused, anxious, disempowered, and on the verge of giving up. Is pain a complete mystery?

Unfortunately, the heroine in our back pain story represents a very common case, one that plays out thousands of times per day across the country. Most people in her situation are never provided with the knowledge and education that could help them make sense of their condition, and make the most intelligent and empowering choices about how to manage it. My intention with this chapter is to help remedy that problem.

The study of pain has advanced a great deal in the last fifty years, but unfortunately it has been slow to have an impact on the way pain is commonly treated. Much of what has been learned is surprising and counterintuitive. And it is very consistent with the primary theme of this book — that the source of physical dysfunction is sometimes located more in the nervous system than the body.

A paradigm shift in understanding pain: the neuromatrix

An excellent way to understand the findings of pain science is the neuromatrix model, developed by Ronald Melzack and Patrick Wall, and further popularized by David Butler and Lorimer Moseley.[64] The neuromatrix helps explain the relationship between pain, tissue damage, sensory signaling, perception, movement, thought, and emotion.

The "neuromatrix" sounds like an intimidating concept, but it simply means the patterns of brain activity that create pain.[65] Just as there is a particular pattern of brain activity or "neurotag" that creates the conscious experience of tasting chocolate, seeing the color blue, or being touched on the hand, there is also a particular neurotag for all the varieties of pain that you experience. When you hit yourself on the thumb with a hammer, there is a certain pain neurotag that creates that special feeling. If you hit yourself on the thumb and for some reason this does *not* activate a pain neurotag, you will *not* feel pain in the thumb. And if for some reason your thumb pain neurotag is activated, *even if you haven't hit your thumb at all,* you will feel pain in the thumb.

Thus, pain is a conscious experience created by the brain, not a damaged condition of the body. You can have one without the other. The experience of phantom limb pain provides a perfect example — even though the limb is gone, the virtual limb remains, and can be activated. You don't need a body to feel a body, and you don't need tissue damage to feel pain.

Pain is for protection

Pain is easier to understand when we consider that its purpose is to motivate protective behaviors. Like other perceptions, pain serves a function: in this case, to protect the body from perceived threat. Like an alarm system in a house, the pain system is set up to detect danger and signal the need for protective action. Further, the sensitivity and volume of the alarm can be turned up and down, depending on the circumstances. We will discuss this in more detail later in this section.

Pain is an output not an input

Another central idea in the neuromatrix model is that pain is an "output" of the brain, not a signal or "input" to the brain from the body.[66] In this sense, the pain alarm system is like the movement system, in that it gathers information from the body, interprets it, and then creates outputs to accomplish goals. With pain, the goal is to encourage behaviors to protect the body from perceived threats.

What are the different kinds of information or "inputs" that contribute to pain? The most important input is usually nociception — sensory signaling indicating danger to the tissues of the body. Given its key role in pain, we will look at the physiology of nociception in more detail in a later section.

But nociception is not the *only* important input. When the brain receives a danger signal from the body, it will need to ask: "how dangerous is this really?" To answer, it draws on every available and credible piece of information related to threat, including other sensory cues, past memories, and emotions. Here are some examples of how inputs other than nociception modulate pain.

Proprioception will alter pain because the brain will recognize certain body positions as indicating danger, and others as being safe. For example, if your shoulder is dislocated, or your back is in the same position as it was during a previous injury, proprioception will report the bad news, which will probably make pain worse.

What you see and hear also provides information relevant to threat, and therefore has a strong power to affect pain. Here's an interesting example: a man was admitted to the emergency room with a nail through his boot. He was in excruciating pain. His pain ceased when removal of the boot revealed the nail had missed his foot and gone between his toes.[67] I assume the man was happy but probably a little embarrassed.

Thoughts and expectations affect pain. If you think that a particular stimulus will cause pain, then pain is more likely.[68] If you are a cancer patient recovering from surgery, your pain is likely to be worse if you think it indicates a return of cancer, as opposed to a natural part of the healing process.[69] Musicians will suffer more pain from a prick to the finger than people who don't care as much about the function of their hands.[70]

Pain researcher Lorimer Moseley tells a humorous story about walking in the desert near a place where he had recently received a near fatal snakebite.[71] While walking, a bush scratched his leg in the same place where he had been previously bitten. He immediately experienced excruciating pain all over his leg. Apparently his brain misinterpreted the scratch as being another bite. In other words, the decisive "input" which produced his pain was a bad memory, not nociceptive signaling.

Emotions are another cognitive input that can have a significant impact on pain. Psychological states associated with depression, anxiety, hopelessness, fear and lack of control are all associated with chronic pain.[72]

Social context is also relevant. Part of the way we protect ourselves from physical harm is getting assistance from others. Therefore, pain can change depending on our perception that we have financial and social support to deal with an injury.[73] If a man has a very caring wife, do you think he will feel more pain when she is *in* the room or *out* of the room? Tough guys are not so tough when someone is there to kiss their owies.

Thus, our movements, thoughts, emotions, and memories all have an effect on pain. Although nociception is one of the most important inputs contributing to pain, it is neither necessary nor sufficient for pain to exist. We can have pain without nociception, and nociception without pain.

Here is a very important point of clarification: *none of this means that pain is not real, or that it is all in your head*. Pain is real. Pain is a real *feeling*, but that feeling does not necessarily reflect real damage in the body. Further, although pain depends on brain activity for its existence, this does not mean you can simply think pain away or that pain is your fault. Unfortunately, the processes which create pain are mostly unconscious and outside your control. Although your conscious thoughts about pain can change it, the effects are in many cases small.

With that caveat in mind, let's take a closer look at some of the above ideas in more detail.

Pain Does Not Equal Tissue Damage

It is generally true that the more your body is damaged, the more pain you will feel. But there is not a one-to-one relationship there, and sometimes there is a major divergence. In other words, there are many cases where people experience significant injury without pain, or extreme pain with little or no injury. Pain without damage is particularly common in cases of chronic pain.

Tissue damage without pain

Dramatic examples of extreme harm without pain may occur when a soldier is wounded in battle, or a surfer gets an arm bit off by a shark. In these situations, there is a good chance the victim will not feel *any* pain until the emergency is over. Have you ever seen an athlete sustain a severe injury on the sports field but not show any signs of pain? (If you only watch soccer, probably not. The reverse is quite likely though.)

Common examples of tissue damage without pain are provided by the numerous studies involving MRI examination of joints that are *not* painful. These consistently show that surprisingly large percentages of people with pain free backs, shoulders, hips and knees have significant damage. Here is a brief survey of some representative studies where MRIs were performed on people with *no* pain.

* **Backs**: Fifty two percent of people with pain free backs had at least one bulging disc or other MRI abnormality.[74] In a similar study, one third of individuals who had never suffered back pain had a substantial spinal abnormality, and 20 percent under the age of sixty had a herniated disc.[75]

* **Hips**: Among pain free hockey players, seventy percent had abnormal pelvis or hip MRIs, and fifty-four percent had labral tears.[76]

* **Knees**: Sixty percent of people with pain free knees, aged twenty to sixty-eight, showed abnormalities in at least three of the four regions of the knee.[77]

* **Shoulders**: In one study, twenty-three percent of people with asymptomatic shoulders had a rotator cuff tear. The authors considered this percentage to be "astonishingly high" and concluded that "rotator cuff tears must to a certain extent be regarded as "normal" degenerative attrition, not necessarily causing pain and functional impairment."[78] In pain free overhead athletes, forty percent of dominant shoulders had findings consistent with partial or full thickness tears of the rotator cuff, as compared with zero percent of the nondominant shoulders. But neither shoulder hurt, and none of the athletes had any pain or problematic symptoms five years after the study.[79]

This is just a small sampling of similar studies, but the pattern is clear. Almost no matter where you point an MRI on an adult body, you can find something wrong there, even parts that are completely free of pain. Degenerative changes in the back, knees, shoulders and every other major joint are normal and predictable parts of life that do not necessarily result in pain.

Pain without tissue damage

On the other end of the spectrum, many people suffer from pain when there is no tissue damage at all. For some, a light touch on the hand can cause excruciating pain. And people with phantom limbs can have pain in a limb that is not even there.

In more common experience, most low back pain is classified as non-specific — it cannot be attributed to any known pathology in the back. In other words, as far as we know, the structure and health of the backs of most people with chronic low back pain is not different from pain free individuals.

So why does chronic pain correlate poorly with the objective state of the body parts that are in pain? Why is pain not an accurate indicator of tissue damage? Here are two reasons.

First, the purpose of pain is not to measure tissue damage, but to encourage protective behaviors. The need for protection depends on more than just the state of the tissues. Second, pain protects against "perceived" threat, not actual threat, and the brain's perceptions in this regard can simply be incorrect. Let's look at these two factors in more detail below.

Pain is an Action Signal Not a Damage Meter

Recall from the previous chapter that our perceptions about body position are created for a purpose — to assist the performance of functional goals. We don't just perceive everything that is there to be perceived. We see what is useful to see, hear what is useful to hear, and have kinesthetic awareness of the body to the extent that it facilitates useful movements.

Similarly, the conscious experience of pain doesn't exist just to let you know a body part is damaged. It is there to motivate protective behaviors such as withdrawing from a noxious stimulus, avoiding movements that aggravate damage, and seeking support and care from others. Thus, *pain is an action signal, not a damage meter.*[80]

When no action is necessary, or action has already been taken, pain serves less of a purpose, and we can expect that in these situations, pain will be less likely, even if there is tissue damage. Here are some examples.

Emergencies

As noted above, soldiers in the course of battle often don't experience pain from severe injuries. The likely explanation is that the protective behaviors encouraged by pain would impair chances of survival. Have you ever received an injury during a competition that you didn't even notice until hours after the game?

When healing is complete

One of the purposes of pain is to allow time to heal from injury. What if time has passed and the injury has healed to the greatest extent possible? Even if some damage persists, your nervous system might conclude the injury is not going to get any better and further protective action is more trouble than it is worth.

This might be the case in regard to damage that is effectively permanent, such as degenerative changes to joints. The damage accumulated slowly over a long period of time, and then healed to the best extent possible. In this circumstance, pain serves less of a purpose.

Placebos: when corrective action has been taken

The placebo effect describes the reduction of pain by the mere expectation that a certain intervention will work, as opposed to making substantive changes in the areas targeted for treatment.[81] This effect is easy to understand when we think of pain as an action signal.

Here is an analogy to illustrate, based on thirst and dehydration. The purpose of thirst is to motivate you to drink water to protect against the perceived threat of dehydration. The thirst will end as soon as you drink what the brain thinks is an adequate amount of water. The interesting thing is that *thirst ends before the tissues are actually rehydrated.* So, even as your tissues continue to signal your brain about their dehydrated state, this does not result in feeling any thirst, because your brain believes that any threat related to dehydration has already been remedied. The brain is essentially saying: "Okay, I hear there's dehydration in the body, but we just drank some water. Help is on the way, and therefore, we won't be creating any thirst to encourage protective action in the form of drinking."

Many researchers and clinicians believe a similar logic underlies the efficacy of many placebo treatments. A pill is given, a needle is inserted, a trip to the doctor is made, and the brain concludes that help is on the way, that protective action has been taken, and that pain is no longer necessary, even as the body continues to signal the presence of tissue damage.[82] We'll discuss some of the mechanisms by which this might occur in the next section on nociception.

Pain Protects Against Perceived Threat, Not Actual Threat

Like other perceptions, the perception of threat can be inaccurate. Once again, phantom limb pain provides the perfect example of the brain making a mistake about the existence of threat. There are many other more common-place instances where the brain does not know what is going on in the body, and causes pain in an area that is clearly not under threat.

Any kind of referred pain, where pain is felt a distance from the actual problem, is an example of this. When someone has a heart attack, they will often feel extreme pain in the left arm as opposed to the heart. This might be because the nerves that transmit information about the heart enter the spine very close to nerves coming from the left arm. Because the spine rarely receives any danger signals from the heart, it misinterprets the information as coming from the left arm. So pain is "referred" from the heart to the arm.

People who suffer from allodynia experience pain in response to innocu-ous stimuli such as a light touch. This happens because the mechanoreception that results from the touch is "misread" by the spinal cord as nociception. The brain creates pain in the hand because it believes there is threat there, even though there is none. It is a simple case of miscommunication.

We'll get more into the mechanics of how these miscommunications might happen later, but for now it is sufficient to understand that information processing about threat is an imperfect process that does not always result in the brain knowing exactly what is going on where.

Inputs and Outputs: An Example

Now that we've discussed the basics of how the pain alarm system pro-cesses inputs and produces outputs, let's use an example to illustrate. Consider someone who bends over to pick something up and feels some pain. What are the relevant inputs into the neuromatrix, or pain alarm system? Here is one possible scenario.

The forward bend creates a minor degree of mechanical damage that triggers nociceptors in the low back, which report danger to the brain. This prompts the brain to ask: how dangerous is this really? To answer, it will consider all credible and relevant sources of information.

Proprioceptive, vestibular and visual information report the positions of all the different body parts and whether they are controlled and balanced. They provide information showing that balance is very poor and that a fall may be coming. The brain maps for perceiving the back are fuzzy and there is not a clear picture of where the back is and what it is doing. This confusion contributes to a sense of threat.

The part of the brain that stores memories reports this is the exact same position the body was in last year when it experienced extreme back pain that lasted for several weeks. Another part of the brain remembers a statement by a doctor about a "slipped disc." Another part recognizes that he may be unable to do his job, and that he will need to file for worker's compensation. This immediately causes emotions of intense worry and anxiety about the future, and thoughts of catastrophe.

All these inputs are instantly processed and filtered and analyzed and integrated unconsciously in the brain, which will then ask essentially two questions. How dangerous is this really, and is pain necessary for protection? The resulting pain depends on how the questions are answered.

Are you skeptical that your brain could think this fast, and without you being aware of any of it? Recall the optical illusion with the checkerboard. In interpreting the meaning of the light bouncing off the board, your brain instantaneously took account of the alternating color pattern and the existence of the shadows. The pain alarm system involves just as much unconscious calculation and interpretation as the visual system.

Now consider another person who does the same forward bend, suffers the exact same mechanical damage and resulting nociception, but has a completely different set of proprioceptive and cognitive inputs.

This person moves with good balance, has no memory of any previous back pain, is not afraid of back injury, knows from pain education that back pain does not necessarily imply tissue damage, has excellent financial and social support and is optimistic about the future. Will this person have the same kind of pain? Probably not!

And to further illustrate the complexity and individuality of pain, let's remember that pain is not the only "output" the brain can choose to protect the body. It can choose between several other kinds of protective outputs, such as movements (flinching, limping, muscle guarding, stiffness), autonomic changes (fight or flight), or immune responses (e.g. inflammation). Or some combination of all three in varying amounts.

Further, any output will immediately become a new input into the system. For example, a protective movement will modify the proprioceptive inputs to the brain. Pain will create new thoughts, feelings, and knowledge about dangers to the body. Inflammation will sensitize nociceptors. And so new outputs are created which immediately become inputs again.

The point is that this is an incredibly complex and dynamic system that loops back on itself every second in an unpredictable and inherently personal and individualized manner. Pain is rarely simple!

Now that we have a broad overview of the purpose of pain, its relationship to tissue damage, and how it encourages protective behaviors, let's look at the physiology of how the pain alarm system works. We will start with danger detection in the periphery, communication of danger signals to the spinal cord, relay of these danger signals from the spinal cord up to the brain, and then processing of this information in the brain.

Here is fair warning before you get started with the following section: it is a little bit on the technical side!

If this is not your area of interest and you prefer to skip to the end of this chapter to get some big picture takeaways and practical advice, go ahead and skip to the Summary. But if you are fascinated by the scientific details (It is fascinating!), read ahead.

Here's another good reason to review this section: it encourages respect for the complexity of the pain alarm system.

If you asked five economists to identify the cause of a fiscal crisis, and prescribe a solution, you might get five completely different answers. That is because the economic system involves the complex interactions of millions of different moving parts, and there is imperfect data about the state of each variable. Similarly, if you ask five professionals who treat pain about why a certain patient has chronic back pain, you might get five completely different diagnoses and prescriptions. Again, that is because we are dealing with a complex system and imperfect information about all the relevant variables. If you or anyone else thinks they know *exactly* why something hurts and *exactly* what needs to be done about it, the information in this section might make you think twice.

The Physiology of Nociception

Nociception means the transmission of sensory information about noxious stimuli from the body to the brain. We can think of nociception as the process of detecting danger and sending danger signals to the brain. It proceeds through several stages as described below.

Primary nociception: detection of danger

Nociception is initiated by nociceptors, which are sensory receptors on free nerve endings located throughout the body. Nociceptors detect changes in mechanical, thermal, or chemical stimuli.

The mechanical sensors detect pressure changes. They will be triggered when you are cut, struck or pinched. Chemical nociceptors sense changes in local chemistry, which may be caused by inflammation, adrenaline, bursting of cell walls, or an acidic state caused by excess muscle work. Thermal nociceptors detect changes in temperature.[83]

Peripheral sensitization

Nociceptors can change their threshold for firing and their rate of firing by a number of mechanisms. The most common is the presence of inflammation, which lowers the threshold and increases firing rate. This is called peripheral sensitization and it causes hyperalgesia — when a stimulus is more painful than normal. Anti-inflammatory drugs reduce pain by decreasing the inflammation that causes this sensitivity.[84] Stingrays cause pain by doing the opposite — sensitizing nociceptors. If you read accounts of what it feels like to get stung, you will hear some poetic explanations. One victim described the pain as "grinding combined with tearing of the flesh." Sensitization is a powerful thing!

Secondary nociception: danger signals reach the spinal cord

After a nociceptive signal is initiated at the free nerve endings, it travels up the nerve to its end point near the spine, where it communicates over a synapse with the dorsal horn of the spinal cord.[85]

When nociceptive signals reach the end of the nerve, chemicals are released into the synapse that will excite the dorsal horn. When the dorsal horn reaches a threshold level of excitement, it sends a nociceptive signal up the spinal cord to the brain. This is called secondary nociception.[86]

We can think of the dorsal horn as a way station or gate that receives information about danger and then decides if it should be reported to the brain.

Central sensitization: same danger, more danger signals

Like primary nociception, the threshold for activation of secondary nociception in the dorsal horn can be changed — a lot. This has a major effect on pain. As discussed below, it might be the difference between feeling excruciating pain from a light touch, or having your arm cut off and feeling nothing at all.

Recall that when free nerve endings are sensitized, they fire at lower thresholds of stimulation, and this is called peripheral sensitization. Central sensitization occurs when the dorsal horn is sensitized, so that it sends a signal to the brain at lower thresholds of stimulation from free nerve endings.[87]

As with peripheral sensitization, central sensitization can lead to hyperalgesia — more pain than you would normally get from a particular injury. Central sensitization can also cause allodynia — pain from an innocuous stimulus that does not trigger any danger signals at all. This happens when the dorsal horn becomes so sensitive it can be activated by nearby nerves relaying mechanoreceptive information. This "cross-talk" means that a message originally intended to report a light touch or gentle movement is misread by the spinal cord as indicating danger. The result is pain without harm.[88]

Central sensitization is a very normal response to nociceptive signaling from the periphery, and it begins to happen immediately thereafter. Thus, after an injury occurs, the barrage of nociception will quickly sensitize the dorsal horn. Because the dorsal horn receives signals from many peripheral nerves from other areas, the sensitization will be broader than the exact site of damage. This is one of the reasons why pain "spreads" from its original place.[89]

As tissue damage heals and primary nociception is reduced, the sensitivity of the dorsal horn *should* return to baseline levels. However, it appears that some individuals are prone to maintaining sensitization even after tissue damage is healed. This may be a factor explaining why some people develop chronic pain after an injury. For these people, sensitivity can be maintained by far less nociception than what was required to create it in the first place.[90] Pain becomes like a habit that is hard to break.

This is one of the reasons why with chronic pain, the problem might be more about how the nervous system is reporting and processing information and less about whether the body is damaged. If you have pain that has gone on for more than three months, there have definitely been changes in the way your nervous system processes danger signals from the painful area.

Ectopic nociception: danger signals from nerve trunks

Ectopic nociception occurs when nociceptive signals originate from the "wrong place" — the middle of a nerve trunk as opposed to the nerve ending. This may occur as a result of injury or mechanical stress to the connective tissue sheath of the nerve, which causes inflammation.[91]

Inflammation of the connective tissue sheath of a nerve can create spontaneous signal firing from the nerve trunk. The spinal cord will read the signal as coming from the nerve *ending*, not the middle of the trunk, which means pain will be felt some distance from the actual problem. Ectopic firing will also cause a nerve impulse to be sent "down" to the nerve ending (an "antidromic impulse") which will secrete inflammatory chemicals that cause peripheral sensitization near the nerve ending. This is called neurogenic inflammation.[92]

This means inflammation of a nerve trunk can result in a cascade of undesirable events, including ectopic nociception (which helps create central sensitization), and neurogenic inflammation (which creates peripheral sensitization). **It may be a major player in pain that persists, spreads and changes location.**

Descending modulation: changing the volume on nociception

Recall that the dorsal horn is the gateway that reports nociceptive information to the brain. The brain can reduce or increase the sensitivity of this gateway. This is called descending modulation.[93] It is like turning the volume knob up or down on nociceptive signaling. Lorimer Moseley views descending modulation as a way for the brain to "second-guess" the periphery about the threat posed by a particular stimulus.

For example, even though an injury creates only minor nociception, the brain may decide the problem is actually quite serious. In this event, it might use descending modulation to sensitize the dorsal horn and facilitate the transmission of nociceptive signals to the brain. For example, if the brain can see that a knife is sticking into the painful area, or remembers the same area had previously sustained serious injury, it might sensitize the area. In fact, research shows if you expect a particular stimulus to be painful, this will increase the level of nociceptive firing in the spinal cord.[94] This is an example of a "nocebo" — when thoughts can make pain worse. (Remember the guy with the nail in his boot?)

On the other hand, the brain could use descending modulation to *inhibit* nociception. This might occur when the nociception results from an activity the brain considers desirable or healthy, such as vigorous exercise, a deep tissue massage, or movements that are assisting to escape an emergency. In this event, the brain does not want to discourage the activity that is creating the nociception, and therefore decides to simply block the danger signals.

Descending inhibition may be the mechanism that explains why many people do not feel pain from degenerative changes in joints, bulging discs, or torn rotator cuffs. It also likely explains why pain is often not felt during an emergency.

Descending inhibition is accomplished by what David Butler calls the "the drug cabinet in the brain."[95] There is significant research showing that descending inhibition is not working properly in many chronic pain conditions such as fibromyalgia, irritable bowel syndrome, and TMJ.[96]

Interestingly, descending inhibition is reliably triggered by sustained nociceptive input. Researchers study it by immersing a hand in cold water. Which hurts. This will lead to greater pain tolerance not just from the local area, but distant areas as well. The effectiveness of descending inhibition in suppressing pain is highly dependent on the *expectation* that the stimulus will reduce pain.[97]

This dynamic of fighting pain in one area by creating it in another likely explains the success of many therapies, and is sometimes called counterirritation. The feeling of "good pain" during exercise, a stretch, deep pressure from massage, trigger point work, or foam rolling is a sign the brain is interpreting the noxious stimulus as somehow beneficial, and creating some feel good chemicals to make it more tolerable. The effect is temporary of course.

All these facts imply that the brain's opinions about the meaning of a particular stimulus help determine how it gets processed even at the spinal cord level. In the next section we will discuss how danger signals get processed in the brain.

How the Brain Creates Pain

When nociceptive signals reach the brain, many different parts of the brain become involved in interpreting its meaning and creating an appropriate protective response. Although there are certain areas of the brain that are more active in this process than others, there is no "pain center." Instead, the neural activity associated with pain is widely distributed throughout many areas.[98]

As discussed earlier, the diverse brain areas involved in creating pain are sometimes called the neuromatrix, and the specific pattern of brain activity that generates a particular pain experience has been termed a "neurotag."

The neurotag concept helps illustrate two common problems with chronic pain:

1. Pain neurotags can get facilitated, or easier to activate, so pain thresholds are lowered.

2. Pain neurotags can become "imprecise" due to uncontrolled neuronal activity, and this creates pain in places it doesn't belong.

These two ideas help explain some unusual phenomena we see with persistent pain — how it can spread, change locations, come and go at odd times, and otherwise act like it has a "mind of its own." [99]

Facilitation of pain neurotags: lowered pain thresholds

One way a pain neurotag (or any neurotag) can become facilitated is simply repeated use. Just as you can develop habits of movement by repeatedly activating the neural pathways for that movement, you can develop habits of pain through repetition. The more times you feel a certain pain, the more you will "deepen" the neural grooves that create it, and the less stimulus will be required to trigger it.[100]

Another way a pain neurotag can be facilitated is by excitement of another neurotag that tends to trigger it. This is again related to the concept that neurons that "fire together, wire together."

Let's say you injure your shoulder so that every time you raise your arm overhead, you create nociception and pain. After a while, your brain will strongly associate the movement with pain — the neurotags for the movement and the pain have fired simultaneously so many times they are now "wired" together. If the injury heals and nociception dissipates, the movement might still create pain because of the strong connection in the brain.[101]

This same dynamic explains why pain can be modified by so many inputs. Think of all the associations your brain makes with pain — perhaps a work environment, a social context, a movement or activity, even sights, sounds or ideas. If you experience back pain every day at work for years, you will probably lower your threshold for that pain just by showing up. Most people probably associate the idea of a "slipped disc" with back pain. (Put another way, their neurotags share many "member cells.") Thus, if you think about a slipped disc, you will lower your threshold for back pain. An extreme example of the power of thought to affect pain comes from people who suffer from complex regional pain syndrome. They can experience pain in their affected limb by simply thinking about moving it.[102]

Imprecise neurotags: pain spreads

Excited neurons tend to excite other neurons, unless the spread of excitement is inhibited. Proper inhibition is what creates a meaningful pattern of neural activity, as opposed to an undifferentiated explosion of neural activity like an epileptic seizure. Chronic pain is often related to "disinhibition" — a failure of the inhibitory process. This allows imprecise firing of neurons outside the desired neurotag.[103] Imprecision is one reason why chronic pain can spread beyond the area of actual tissue damage, move from one area to another, or become more difficult to locate in a specific area.

Similar problems with imprecision can affect neurotags for any kind of brain output, including perceptions, thoughts, immune responses and movements. Thus, imprecision is behind a variety of neurological disorders such as bipolar disorder, schizophrenia, Parkinson's disease, dystonia, migraine, and chronic pain.[104]

The importance of accurate maps

We said in an earlier chapter that accurate body maps are necessary for good perception of body position and movement. It appears the accuracy of the maps may also be a factor in chronic pain.

People with chronic pain have been shown to have difficulty in various tasks that require good perception of body location and motor control, including:[105]

* Locating the outline of the back and the position of the spine

* Two-point discrimination

* Right/left discriminations of pictures of body parts

* Reducing postural sway in response to disturbance

* Control of the pelvis and low back

Further, there is evidence that chronic pain patients have changes in brain structure in areas that control perception and movement.

This raises a key question: are problems with perception and movement causing pain, or is pain causing problems with perception and movement?

There is at least some evidence that the relationship is a two way street, and that the interaction between perception and pain is extremely dynamic and complex. Part of the evidence comes from research studying the use of illusions to modulate perception and pain.

Body sense affects body health

The brain helps ensure the physical health of the body by monitoring and regulating almost every aspect of its physiology: temperature, PH, blood flow, hunger, immune responses, hormone levels, etc. But the brain's ability to properly regulate the body will only be as good as its ability to form clear pictures about what is actually going on in the body. As described below, when the brain makes mistakes in mapping the position of the body, there are some very interesting effects.

One aspect of mapping the body we probably take for granted is knowledge about which physical objects are part of the body and which are not. But the sense of "ownership" is not a given. It is fairly easy to encourage the brain to take ownership over inanimate objects, and "neglect" actual body parts. One of the best ways to cause this confusion is with the rubber hand illusion, which works as follows.

One hand is placed on a table, the other out of sight behind a screen. A rubber hand is placed to the side of the hand that remains in sight. The subject's hand behind the screen is then stroked with a brush while he watches the rubber hand stroked in the same way. Pretty soon he will get an uncanny sense that the rubber hand is part of his body, and he will even flinch when it is threatened.

This means the brain takes "ownership" of the rubber hand. Even more interesting is the brain also disowns or "neglects" the hand that is out of sight. *We know this because the hand behind the screen actually gets colder, the result of a change in blood flow.*[106] Thus, mapping errors affect blood flow. They also affect immune responses: a hand that has been disowned through use of the rubber hand illusion will suffer more inflammation in response to a physical insult than a normal hand.[107] These are truly remarkable findings. They show our brain's sense of self directly affects its physiological regulation.

Further, neglect of body parts is not something that happens only in highly artificial conditions created by illusions. People with chronic back pain have trouble perceiving the outline of their back.[108] Patients with CRPS suffer neglect of their affected hand. They also neglect the *space* around the hand, so that switching hand positions will make the unaffected hand colder.[109] So the brain maps not only body parts, but also the space around the body parts, and the map affects any body part in that space.[110] This shows our sense of self is highly complex and can be modified in ways that are hard to imagine and that make a difference.

Sensory motor mismatch: bad predictions cause pain

Whenever the brain makes a movement, it predicts the sensory information that will result. The predicted feedback is compared to determine if the movement was successful. If the sensory data consistently conflicts with the prediction, this is called sensory motor mismatch.

It stands to reason that sensory motor mismatch is more likely to occur when the body maps are smudged or inaccurate. Some researchers believe confusion resulting from sensory motor mismatch can cause perception of threat, and this plays a role in certain chronic pain conditions. In fact, research shows that artificially induced sensory motor mismatch can make pain worse in chronic pain patients, and that correcting the mismatch can alleviate the pain.

You can create sensory motor mismatch in the following way. Place your arms on either side of a mirror so the right arm is behind the mirror and the left arm is in front. Look at the reflection of the stationary left arm while moving the right arm that is hidden behind the mirror. This creates confusion because the brain sees what looks like the right arm as being stationary, but feels it moving. It is not surprising this would feel weird, but it can also cause pain. In one study, twenty-six of twenty-nine fibromyalgia patients performing this activity reported feeling a transient increase in pain or other symptoms indicating a flare-up of their condition.[111]

Studies on the thermal grill illusion provide further evidence that sensory-motor mismatch can cause pain, *and* that correcting it can reduce pain. The thermal grill illusion involves placing the index and ring fingers in warm water and the middle finger in cold water. This unusual sensory input apparently confuses the brain into thinking the middle finger is in painfully hot water, because that is how it feels.

In a recent study, researchers induced pain through the TGI and asked the subjects to press their fingers together.[112] This cut pain levels by 64 percent. However, they were unable to reduce the pain by doing several other forms of touching, such as touching the hands of other people, or by pressing their hands together in an overlapping fashion. In other words, the pain didn't go away until the brain received sensory information to correct the mismatch.

Another study indicating that correction of sensory motor mismatch can reduce chronic pain involves people with low back pain making certain provocative movements of their back.[113] Watching the movements in a mirror makes the movements less painful. Perhaps this is because the visual information corrects errors in sensory feedback caused by poor mapping of the movement. Seeing it helps.

❋ Summary

The science on pain is fascinating, counterintuitive, and somewhat mind-boggling. It is easy to get blown away by all the details and strangeness of pain. However, there are a few simple takeaways from all this information that I will discuss in this section. And there are even fewer common sense practical suggestions that I will discuss in the section that immediately follows.

* Pain is a conscious experience that requires a certain pattern of brain activity for its existence. The neuromatrix is the pattern of brain activity, that when activated, creates pain.

* Without the activation of a pain neurotag, there will be no pain, even if the body is damaged. If a pain neurotag is activated, there will be pain, even if the body is not damaged at all.

* Nociception is neither sufficient nor necessary for pain. Instead, it is just one of many inputs into the pain alarm system. Cognitive and proprioceptive inputs also modulate pain.

* The purpose of pain is to motivate protective behaviors, not act as a reflection of reality. Thus, pain is an action signal, not a measurement of damage.

* Although pain is the result of brain activity, and thoughts modulate pain, pain is not "in your head." We cannot just think pain away by changing our thoughts, because a great deal of the brain activity that creates pain is unconscious and non-voluntary.

* There is not a one-to-one correlation between tissue damage and pain. Many people without pain show significant damage on MRIs. On the other hand, many chronic pain conditions are characterized by hyperalgesia and/or allodynia, where stimuli that are normally non-painful cause pain.

* Pain is based on perception of threat. The processes that relay information about danger from the periphery to the brain are subject to error and miscommunication. Thus, pain can be referred to an area that is not damaged, or innocuous sensory signals about movement can be misinterpreted by the spinal cord as nociceptive signals.

* Nociception is the transmission of sensory information about noxious stimuli from the periphery to the brain. Primary nociception occurs at free nerve endings. Ectopic nociception occurs in nerve trunks that are inflamed. Secondary nociception occurs at the dorsal horn of the spinal cord.

* Peripheral sensitization lowers the firing threshold for the free nerve endings. Central sensitization lowers the threshold of the dorsal horn. Descending modulation from the brain modifies the sensitivity of the dorsal horn. Together, these factors turn the volume up or down on nociception.

* Pain neurotags are facilitated through repetition. They can also become "wired" to other neurotags (e.g. for movement) if they frequently fire simultaneously.

* The failure to inhibit the unwanted spread of neural activation can be termed imprecision or disinhibition. Pain neurotags are subject to disinhibition, imprecision, or smudging, which can result in the unwanted spread of pain.

* The accuracy of the body maps affects the homeostatic and physiological regulation of the body.

∗ Chronic pain is associated with imprecise body maps and poor performance on tasks requiring proprioceptive acuity or body sense. Sensory motor mismatch may be a mechanism for chronic pain. Correcting it may be a treatment.

Common Mechanisms for Pain Relief

So what can we do with all this information? Based on the science discussed in this chapter, following are some common mechanisms by which different movement practices or manual therapies could be expected to reduce pain.

First, a word of caution. Reading the strategies below is no substitute for getting medical attention. Make sure to see a qualified medical professional for treatment of any pain.

Reducing nociception

The most obvious and commonly used strategy for treatment of pain is to find and eliminate sources of nociception near the area that hurts. This might be done through altering biomechanics, trying to get rid of trigger points, reducing excess muscle tension, freeing restrictions on healthy nerve movement, avoiding provocative movements, getting surgery, etc. This strategy is so obvious it almost goes without saying, but it bears mention for a couple reasons.

First, many pain interventions begin and end with this strategy while ignoring others. That is unfortunate.

Second, it is often assumed that when a treatment is effective at reducing pain, it worked by reducing nociception. Because pain is modulated by many factors, this is an invalid assumption that leads to confusion. For example, just because you feel better after massage or acupuncture or stretching doesn't mean that what you did corrected any damage in the tissues.

Third, identifying an exact source of nociception and determining an effective remedy is often *very* difficult. There are many tough questions. Is the source of nociception mechanical or chemical? Are the signals resulting from damage to muscles, tendons, ligaments, fascia, viscera or nerves? Do the signals originate from a nerve ending or a nerve trunk? Is there sensitization peripherally or centrally? What is the role of descending influences?

Is inflammation a significant player and why is it there? Answering these questions is far beyond the scope of this book, and requires significant training and expertise. But just knowing the questions exist is a way to protect against overconfidence and unwarranted assumptions in diagnosing the origin of nociception in any particular case.

Thus, although finding and reducing nociception should be a primary goal of any attempt to reduce pain, it will often require individualized analysis and treatment from a skilled expert. And, despite best efforts, the result will often be frustration. *By contrast, many of the pain relief strategies described below, most of which target inputs aside from nociception, are relatively easy to apply, and are likely to benefit a wide range of conditions and people.* In fact, they are probably sufficient to explain most of the results seen in most therapies, most of which mistakenly claim to work by reducing nociception!

Avoiding painful movements

Avoiding painful movement is an obvious way to treat pain: if it hurts don't do it! But this simple rule receives added support from an understanding of pain science. Sustained nociceptive input can sensitize the nervous system, both peripherally and centrally. Pain could become a *habit*. Thus, repeated provocative movements might make pain worse and last longer, even if they are not causing progressive tissue damage. With this in mind, avoiding a painful movement for some period of time can be a strategy to prevent or break a pattern of sensitivity.

This strategy is often ignored in cases where the pain is just mild or annoying. For example, your back might hurt a little every time you bend forward, or maybe your foot hurts every time you run, but not enough to encourage you to stop engaging in these movements or find a different way to do them.

But these same movements, if repeated often enough, might be sufficient to maintain or increase unwanted sensitization. In these cases, a conscious strategy of "pain starvation" may help break a vicious cycle. This strategy might involve altering the biomechanics of a painful movement, or just avoiding the movement altogether for a while. Of course, avoiding movement could have negative effects if it leads to excessive fear of movement, impairment of function, or deconditioning.

Graded exposure

Graded exposure is the progressive introduction of threatening movements or other stimuli, in the appropriate dosage and timing, in a way that causes the nervous system to become *less* threatened by the movements.[114] The simple rationale is that if you successfully and painlessly perform a movement that used to hurt, your nervous system will find that movement less threatening in the future. We can look at graded exposure as a plan for "threat inoculation."

Any form of vigorous movement that does not cause pain is a potential form of graded exposure, because it gives the brain good news about the health and capacity of the body. This reduces threat and pain, and helps explain why general exercise often performs just as well as many specific interventions for chronic pain, such as core stability work or stretching.[115]

Graded exposure often involves using creativity to find an alternative way to painlessly perform a movement that is normally painful. This can help break unwanted connections in the brain between movement and pain neurotags. This strategy is discussed in more detail later in this book.

Pain science education

Research shows that learning about pain physiology improves chronic pain.[116] Why? From the neuromatrix perspective, education changes cognitive inputs, which modify the output of pain. Education in pain science is a way to correct unsupported ideas about pain that increase threat unnecessarily, and cause people to avoid movement and exercise that is healthy. Such ideas are rampant. For example, many people believe that:

* Their knee is "bone on bone"

* They have the "neck of a ninety-year-old"

* Their back is "out"

* Their herniated disc looks like one of those plastic spinal models with a bulging red blob coming out

* Their pain will never get better and they are powerless to change it

Pain education can dispel these myths and neutralize unnecessary anxiety and fear of movement that will only make pain worse.

Although pain education has been demonstrated to be effective as a way to reduce pain, it is by no means a cure. Conscious knowledge that an area is not actually damaged will not necessarily alter the brain's opinion about the area.

Refinement of motor sensory maps

Working to improve the accuracy of the motor sensory maps may help with chronic pain.[117] We want to make sure our maps are as clear and accurate as possible, so the brain does not mistakenly put pain somewhere it doesn't belong, mistake normal sensory information for pain signaling, or otherwise just become threatened by the fact that it doesn't really know where the body is or how to move it well.

In fact, research shows physical therapy interventions that focus on improving motor control are generally the most effective methods for treating chronic low back pain.[118] The lessons at the end of this book discuss motor control strategies in more detail.

Sensory gating

Sensory gating means the processing and perception of sensory information is reduced by the presence of other competing sense information.[119] If your nervous system is busy trying to process signals resulting from movement or touching, it has less ability to process nociception.

You have probably instinctively taken advantage of sensory gating by rubbing an area that has just been injured. It appears sensory gating and resulting pain relief will be greater where:

* The competing stimulus is closer to the area of pain

* The competing stimulus is more interesting and novel

* The stimulus comes from active movement rather than passive movement or touching

Sensory gating is probably one of the major reasons people feel better after exercise or bodywork. Although the pain killing effects of sensory gating are likely to be temporary, they open a window of opportunity to gain more lasting benefits of performing movements that are normally painful.

Counterirritation

Counterirritation is a way to induce descending inhibition of nociception. This is probably a common mechanism for pain relief in therapies that involve a painful stimulus, such as:

* Intense stretches

* Foam rolling

* Trigger point work

* Instrument assisted soft tissue manipulation

* Deep tissue massage.

Creating pain to treat pain may be a risky strategy: getting aggressive can make pain worse not better, or even cause an injury. With this in mind, it may be best to ensure that any pain resulting from therapy feels like a "good pain." This may be a sign the nervous system interprets the stress of the treatment to be healthy.

As with sensory gating, temporary pain relief can be a window of opportunity in which to engage in movements that are normally painful and reduce threat associated with those movements.

Emotions

Emotions affect pain. If you are feeling stressed, anxious, depressed, pessimistic, powerless and victimized, this will probably make your pain worse. Therefore, anything that can be done to improve your emotional state in a positive direction is something that may improve pain.

Improve general health

Although this book focuses on solutions to pain that are based on the way the nervous system controls movement and perception, it needs to be remembered that anything that promotes general health may help with pain. Eating better, sleeping better, reducing stress, having healthy relationships, finding a sense of meaning in life, and engaging in healthy exercise are all crucial elements in reducing pain, as well as obtaining any other health benefit. Better movement is only one piece of the puzzle!

CHAPTER 6

MOVEMENT AND THREAT: CENTRAL GOVERNORS

"The sense of fatigue is often a very fallacious index of the working capacity of the body. There is not necessarily any correspondence between the subjective feelings of fatigue and the capacity of the muscles to perform work. It is a protective feeling which tends to restrain the man from continuing to perform muscular work when this would cause injury."

— Francis Bainbridge

WE HAVE ALREADY DISCUSSED the idea that pain is a protective output of the nervous system in response to a perceived threat. There are many other ways for the nervous system to protect the body without using pain. In this section we will discuss several ways the nervous system can protect us from movements, especially powerful movements that might cause injury. The mechanism is very simple — if the nervous system thinks a particular movement is threatening, it can simply prevent us from making it.

For example, if the nervous system perceives that a maximum effort muscle contraction might create forces that will cause injury, it can limit the neural drive to the muscle, making a full contraction impossible, regardless of conscious intention.

Similar involuntary protective mechanisms may be at play in modifying or governing flexibility, endurance, and coordination patterns. These mechanisms mean that one limiting factor in reaching your physical potential is the extent to which your nervous system is in a protective mode.

Imagine an overprotective mother riding in a car with her teenage son, and putting her foot on the brake whenever she thinks he is driving unsafely. The speed of the car would be limited not by how much horsepower is under the hood, but Mom's perception of danger.

Similarly, your ability to fully express your potential strength, flexibility, endurance and coordination is limited by your brain's perception of threat associated with the chosen movements. We may not consider a sprained ankle or torn hamstring to be really scary, but our nervous systems evolved in an environment when these injuries could mean the difference between life and death. Preventing them is a major concern.

Thus, your brain is always acting as a governor on your performance, to protect you from yourself, ensuring that you do not move too powerfully, too fast, too far, for too long, or with certain movement patterns.

In this section we'll discuss the science behind central governors related to strength, flexibility, endurance and coordination, and how one of the best and quickest ways to increase performance is to reduce perceived threat.

Threat and Strength

Strength is the ability to create force with muscle contraction. High levels of force are useful, but also potentially dangerous. The powerful contractions that allow us to sprint, cut and handle heavy weight can cause injury in the hamstrings, achilles, ACL, rotator cuff, etc.

We can appreciate the destructive power of muscular force by considering the effects of severe electric shock, which causes involuntary maximum muscle contractions. These are so powerful they can dislocate joints, break bones, throw the body across the room, and cause brain injury through huge rises in blood pressure. So the potential strength of our musculature is greater than we might imagine.

Vladimir Zatsiorsky, a professor of kinesiology and exercise science, estimates the average person can voluntarily utilize only about 65 percent of her potential muscle power. A trained power lifter might reach 80 percent.[120] As kettlebell guru Pavel Tsatsouline says, your muscles are already capable of lifting a car, they just don't know it yet. That is a bit of an exaggeration of course, but it is true that most of us have significant untapped potential in our musculature.

One way to tap that potential is to reduce perceived threat associated with force production. This will give the nervous system the "green light" to use maximum force. There are several lines of research that support this view.

First, experimentally induced pain will weaken a muscle, while anesthetic injected into a painful joint will increase strength.[121] Thus, pain seems to have a "red light" effect on muscle force.

Second, temporary strength increases are often seen immediately after interventions that create novel proprioceptive input, such as joint mobilization.[122] Why? Mobilization could reduce nociception through sensory gating, or by temporarily increasing coordination. A coordinated joint is necessarily a safer joint. Just as you wouldn't move quickly in a basement with poor lighting, your brain doesn't want to move joints quickly and powerfully without a good map of the joint.

Third, strength increases as we get more familiar with a movement through repetition. Of course, part of the reason is improved skill in muscle recruitment. But another reason might be graded exposure — safe repetitions signal to the nervous system that the movement is safe. In this sense, we can look at strength training as a form of threat inoculation. Each safe repetition is further evidence the structure of the body can safely handle strong forces. Interestingly, strength is often quite specific. It will not necessarily transfer to an unfamiliar context, which might be perceived as threatening until proven safe.

This information does not imply that strength is "all in your head," or that a ninety-nine pound weakling could perform great feats of strength with the right mindset. (Despite urban legends to the contrary, my research does not reveal any documented cases of grandmothers lifting cars off children in emergencies!)

But it does suggest that reducing threat associated with forceful movements through safe and pain free repetition, and eliminating pain associated with movement, are key ingredients in a strength training program.

Put another way, we can look at weakness as a protective mechanism of the nervous system, and we can reduce the use of that mechanism by reducing perception of threat.

Threat and Flexibility

Like strength, excess flexibility creates the threat of injury. The further a joint moves away from neutral into the end range of motion, the greater the chance for tissue damage, particularly when the movement involves uncontrolled forces. Therefore, we would expect that like strength, the nervous system will involuntarily limit flexibility to ensure safety.

For example, imagine performing a forward bend and trying to put your palms flat on the floor without bending the knees. Your nervous system might fear this movement will damage your hamstrings, or maybe the nerves that run down the back of the leg. To protect you, it will stiffen the hamstrings to prevent you from hurting yourself. In other words, hamstring stiffness is a protective mechanism.

The idea that flexibility is limited by the nervous system is supported by research showing increases in flexibility from stretching are likely caused by increased stretch *tolerance*, rather than increased length of the muscle.[123]

What would make the nervous system more tolerant to stretch? Based on the above reasoning, anything that will reduce perceived threat in regard to range of motion should increase tolerance to stretch.

We would guess the nervous system would be less threatened by end range movements that are familiar, coordinated, pain free and easily reversed back to a neutral position. With this in mind, it is interesting to consider the many stretching techniques that incorporate neurological "tricks," such as PNF, contract/relax, post isometric relaxation, reciprocal inhibition, etc. Looking at these techniques through the lens of the central governor, we can see them as ways to convince the nervous system that the movement is controlled and the muscle is safe. For example, contracting the stretched muscle is a way to show that it has the capability to return the joint to a neutral position.

Activating the antagonist to the stretched muscle shows that the movement is controlled, and part of a useful function. Other movements are a way to map the joint and get familiar in the position.

If you think of the central nervous system as an intelligent and overprotective mother (as opposed to a dumb set of reflexes that can be fooled with some tricks) then you are bound to get the benefit of all the above techniques. And find new ones. Once again, the practical application is any effort to increase flexibility should involve a program of graded exposure and threat inoculation to reduce perception of threat.

Threat and Endurance

According to the central governor model of endurance proposed by researcher Tim Noakes, fatigue is not a physical state of the body, but rather an emotion that is used by the brain to regulate exercise stress.[124] Thus, like pain, fatigue is an output of the brain designed to protect the body.

During exercise, the brain monitors the state of the body and analyzes the threat of injury that might be caused by the energy production systems working beyond their capacity. When threat is deemed to be too high, the brain produces the fatigue that makes continued work undesirable and eventually impossible. So we never really reach our physical limits. The brain shuts things down before that can happen.

Here are some common observations that are explained by the idea of a central governor on endurance:

* Fatigue is affected by the expected duration of exercise

* Athletes run harder in competition than in training

* Athletes speed up at the end of exercise (the end spurt)

* Skeletal muscle is never fully recruited during any form of exercise — 35–50 percent in prolonged exercise and 60 percent during maximal efforts

Further, research shows that fatigue during exercise is affected by a huge variety of factors unrelated to the physical capacity of the muscles, including emotional state, mental fatigue, motivation, self belief, prior knowledge of the duration of exercise, cerebral and arterial oxygenation, muscle glycogen storage, fluid loss, thirst, heat, and more.[125]

Because fatigue is produced by the brain based on its opinions about what is going on in the body, it is subject to error. For example, athletes can be "tricked" into working harder in numerous ways, such as deceiving them about the time or distance they have exercised, cooling hands and palms to fool the brain into thinking core temperature is less elevated, or using a carbohydrate mouth rinse to make the brain think more food energy is on the way. [126]

Again, this does not imply that endurance is all "in your head," or that you could run a record marathon by playing the theme from Rocky on your headphones. The fitness and health of the body is obviously a huge factor in endurance. But the ultimate limiting factor appears to be the brain's willingness to let the body continue to exercise. Of course, the more fit the body is, the more this limit can be extended. But in some cases, there is obviously a divergence between the feeling of fatigue and the actual fitness of the body. Chronic fatigue may be an example of this.

Threat and Motor Control

Altered coordination is another way the central nervous system protects us from perceived threat related to movement. On some level, this should be completely obvious. When our ankle is sprained, we limp. We don't need to consciously choose a new way to walk to protect the ankle. The limp emerges spontaneously and involuntarily.

But compensatory muscle activation patterns can be quite subtle as well. There is a large body of research performed by Paul Hodges and others showing that in the presence of chronic pain, certain muscles, particularly local stabilizers, tend to become delayed in their activation and sometimes atrophied.[127] At the same, global stabilizers tend to get facilitated.

For example, in the presence of back pain, the transversus abdominis and inner obliques tend to get delayed in their activation, while the rectus abdominis and external oblique get facilitated. In the back, the multifidus gets delayed and tends to atrophy, while the erectors increase their activity. With knee pain, the vastus medialis gets inhibited, and in the neck it is the deep neck flexors.[128] As discussed in an earlier section, these are all muscles that fit the local stabilizer category and are ideally suited for creating joint centration.

This raises a very important question. Are these changes in coordination causing the pain? Or is the pain causing the changes in coordination? Or both? The research seems to indicate that pain causes the coordination changes more than vice versa. One persuasive piece of evidence is that characteristic changes in motor coordination and atrophy can be induced experimentally with saline injections to create pain.

According to Hodges, the altered coordination programs are protective in nature.[129] They are caused by interactive changes at multiple levels of the nervous system, including higher levels. Thus, we should view these changes as intelligent and purposeful as opposed to reflexive and random.

How are these changes protective? In general, they prevent movement in painful areas by stiffening them. The mechanical stress of movement is thereby shifted away from the area of pain. While this may be a good short-term strategy, it is often negative in the long-term for several reasons.

For example, in the presence of back pain, the rectus abdominis and erectors increase co-contraction to create more stiffness. This braces the back and protects the painful area, but it comes with a price. Compression is increased, variation in movement is reduced, and there is less ability to make precise intersegmental movements. Thus, co-contraction of the global stabilizers means the back is splinted, but less coordinated and more compressed. It's like wearing an ankle brace — a good short-term strategy for protection, but a poor long-term strategy for function and health. Some movement coaches refer to this bracing as a "high-threshold strategy." Research shows these bracing strategies may continue even after pain has been eliminated.

This research has at least two important implications in regard to efforts to improve coordination. First, the presence of pain will make it very difficult to retrain motor patterns, as the nervous system will tend to involuntarily adopt protective strategies that may be undesirable. Thus, trying to train movement in the presence of threat and pain is very problematic.

Second, areas that are not currently painful may be infected with protective movement patterns that became habitual during a prior episode of pain. Finding and breaking movement habits that involve excess protective muscle stiffness, lack of variability, and poor joint centration may be a worthy goal.

✳ Summary

Protecting the body is one of the main priorities of the central nervous system. Stiffness, weakness, tiredness and altered motor programs are ways for the nervous system to protect us against perceived threats related to movement. Training in the presence of threat will lead to habits of movement and perception that are oriented more toward protection than performance.

Accordingly, one of the quickest and easiest ways to increase performance is to reduce perceived threat related to movement. From this perspective, all methods of training can be thought of as forms of graded exposure or threat inoculation, or a way to send good news to the nervous system about the health and capacity of the body.

CHAPTER 7

MOVEMENT, THINKING AND FEELING

"The hypothesis here to be defended says that this order of sequence is incorrect … that the more rational statement is that we feel sorry because we cry, angry because we strike, afraid because we tremble, and not that we cry, strike, or tremble, because we are sorry, angry, or fearful, as the case may be."
— William James

WE HAVE ALREADY DISCUSSED in previous chapters the close relationship between movement and sense perception. In this section we'll discuss how movement is linked with thought and emotion.

Many movement disciplines such as yoga, dance, martial arts, and the Feldenkrais Method are intended to train the mind through movement of the body. For some practitioners, better movement is not the destination, but instead a vehicle to move forward on a path of discipline, self-discovery, or personal development.

Mindful movement practices can train self-awareness and have a distinctly meditative quality. In fact, many forms of meditation are essentially exercises in focusing attention on the sensations related to the movements of breathing.

The lesson from traditional mind/body practices, and the research summarized in this chapter, is that training the ability to focus attention on information from the body, and to inhibit unwanted movement, may be beneficial to health and emotional well-being on many levels.

Movement and Mood

It is fairly obvious that emotional state affects movement and posture. If you are feeling depressed or submissive, your head may hang. If you are feeling proud or dominant, your chest may rise. This is why we can tell how someone is feeling by his body language.

Some interesting research indicates this relationship works in reverse as well. For example, sitting in an expansive posture, with the arms and limbs out to the sides of the body, will change behavior. It increases dominance, pain tolerance, and risk-taking in a betting game.[130] Sitting in a closed, constricted posture with the limbs inward and touching the body will tend to have opposite effects.

Facial expression also affects mood. Of course we smile when we are happy, but we also get happier if we smile. Thus, holding a pencil between your teeth (which inadvertently puts you in a smiling position) will improve your mood.[131] Botox treatments, which restrict the movement of certain facial muscles, will make it harder to feel the emotions associated with the facial expressions created by those muscles.[132]

There are many other interesting ways in which movements of the body and mental activity interact in surprising ways. Engaging in hand gestures while practicing math leads to quicker learning.[133] Hand washing reduces feelings of guilt.[134] Positive statements are more likely to be accompanied by gestures with the dominant hand than negative statements, which preferentially activate the non-dominant hand.[135] It seems we can't help but associate the wrongness of using the wrong hand with other kinds of wrongness, which is probably why the Italian word for left is sinistra, the French word for left is gauche, and the English and romance language words for right are synonyms for "correct."

This goes to show that the brain's apparently separate outputs are actually very entangled. Moshe Feldenkrais claimed there is no such thing as an isolated emotion, thought, movement or sensation. Each mental output will always involve elements of the other three, so every thought has an associated movement, sensation and emotion; every emotion has a related movement, sensation, and thought, and so on.

For some reason, it is easy for us to understand the connection between thoughts and emotion. Many people will try to "think good thoughts" as a way to change their emotions. But the research suggests that "moving happy moves" might work just as well. As an experiment, next time you are feeling unhappy, try smiling, dancing, or making other movements associated with a more positive mental state. You might hate yourself a little while doing it, but you might also feel a little better immediately afterward.

Motor Control and Emotional Control

As noted in an earlier chapter, skill in movement is largely a matter of inhibition. This is because skill development is characterized not by adding new muscle contractions, but taking away the unnecessary ones.

In the context of everyday emotional life, inhibition allows you to make measured responses to stressful events. When a car cuts you off in traffic, there is a flash of excitement in the muscles and heart rate, but the spread of excitement is (hopefully) quickly inhibited. By contrast, when a two-year-old experiences minor frustration from say, not being able to put on her socks, this could easily magnify into ten minutes of uncontrolled emotional meltdown. The initial excitement spreads like wildfire and can't be controlled.

There are some interesting correlations between poor skill in motor inhibition and increased tendency toward a variety of impulse control disorders. For example, people with ADHD, substance abuse, and gambling addiction perform worse than average on tests of motor inhibition such as a "stop task."[136] (A stop task tests the speed and accuracy of stopping an ongoing movement after a cue.) Based on this and other evidence, many researchers believe the inhibitory mechanisms that control movement are also used to suppress thoughts, emotions and decisions that are potentially harmful.[137]

This is unsurprising because most of our brainpower originally evolved as a way to create movement. Higher order functions such as thought and emotion came later, and had to rely on the previously developed movement software and hardware as a base. Thus, brain areas related to inhibiting motor output also regulate risk-taking behavior. In fact, disruption of a part of the brain responsible for motor planning leads to problems with impulse control and gambling.[138]

Further, it appears that training inhibition skill in movement may improve impulse control in other areas. In one study, people who engaged in a practice requiring movement inhibition took less risks than controls in a subsequent gambling game. The researchers proposed that increased motor cautiousness primed an inhibition system in the brain that regulates a wide range of functions, including impulse control and decision-making. [139]

This is quite interesting because most of the skills we develop are very specific to one particular domain, but useless elsewhere. So it is very good to know which skills are likely to have wide transfer and broad applicability to other domains. In this case, it seems that training motor skills will provide benefits that are not limited to the physical realm. Put simply, it may be that practicing control of movement could help with control of emotion.

Training the Focus of Attention

Another all-purpose mental muscle that may get trained through mindful movement practice is the ability to focus and shift attention. Recall that the brain is constantly filtering sensory information. The direction in which attention is focused will affect what sensory information gets filtered out and what gets processed. In performance, the ability to focus attention is vital to creating the state of deep practice that results in the greatest motor learning.

Is this a trainable skill? There is research suggesting the ability to focus attention is a general skill that is trainable and transferable in various contexts, *including dealing with pain.*

In one study, people trained in an eight-week mindfulness meditation program were better able than controls to shift their attention from their foot to their hand. (This ability to shift attention was measured by alpha wave changes in the brain.)[140]

In another study, students who received meditation training twenty minutes a day for four days experienced approximately half as much pain in response to a constant stimulus when meditating compared to resting.[141] Recent research shows that differences in the brain structures controlling attention are related to sensitivity to pain.[142] Further, multiple randomized clinical trials show strong evidence for the benefit of meditation or mindfulness programs for a wide variety of conditions including chronic pain, fibromyalgia, IBS, depression, and mood disorders.[143] It appears people who are better able to control their attention are also better able to control their pain.

The Right Kind of Attention

Many traditions in mindfulness-based meditation will teach students that when thoughts or emotions arise, the student should resist the impulse to react with emotions or further thoughts. Instead, the thoughts and emotions should be acknowledged in a nonjudgmental way, and attention should be returned to the proper focus — usually the sensory information associated with breathing.

This frame of mind is often referred to as "being present" or "mindful." Researchers sometimes call it "metacognition" — the ability to look at thoughts, perceptions and emotions for what they are — constructions of the brain as opposed to external realities.[144] Metacognition implies not just awareness of what goes on in our heads, but also a nonjudgmental attitude. It is the difference between wise self-knowledge and neurotic self-consciousness.

Applying this skill in the context of movement would imply focusing attention on the sensations of movements, as opposed to any thoughts or judgments you might have about what those sensations mean. For example, in a forward bend, you might be very tempted to start thinking about why your back isn't comfortable. Do I have a herniated disc? Is this related to that old car accident? Are my abs too weak? And does that make my gut look big?

Instead of focusing attention on this type of thinking process, a preferable state of mind would be to simply acknowledge the thoughts, and then return focus to the sensations of the movement. Notice any discomfort, its location, its quality and intensity. But also recognize this is just a feeling about the back that your brain has constructed, not an objective state of the back. And also notice all the other sensations: the feeling of stretching in the hamstrings, the lengthening of the back, the connection of the feet to the floor, the movements of the breath, etc. Taking account of all the sensations, and shifting between them is likely to develop the skills of focusing attention and metacognition that may underlie the benefits of meditation.

If you have done much mindful movement practice, you will probably recognize the benefits of having this type of focused and nonjudgmental attitude as you move. You might have also noticed that after engaging in a particularly mindful session of movement, the benefits spill over to your everyday life. You might find yourself better able to pay close attention to a conversation with a friend, deal with stress, or inhibit unwanted negative emotions. You might feel more "present" and "in the moment." Perhaps this is because your movement practice has primed some general skills in focus of attention and metacognition.

Interoception and Emotion

Although we tend to think our hearts beat faster because we are scared, it is in some ways the reverse. We get scared when we sense through interoception that our heart is beating faster.

Interoception is defined in various ways, but always includes sensory information from the viscera and other organs that indicate the body's physiological state: heart rate, PH, blood pressure, oxygenation of the lungs, fullness of the stomach, etc.

When interoceptive information is interpreted and processed by the brain, the result will be an emotion, feelings of hunger, the need to breathe, anxiety, fear, or arousal.[145] In fact, all emotions are supported and affected by interoceptive information from the body, just as conscious perceptions of hearing and sight are supported by sensory information from the eyes and ears. Thus, fear without a racing heart is not fear. If the body is not moved, neither are the passions.[146]

Research shows that someone's degree of interoceptive awareness can be measured by their ability to detect their own heart rate.[147] Interestingly, people with better interoceptive awareness:

* Experience emotions more strongly, but are also better able to control them

* Are quicker to respond to a painful stimulus, but *less* likely to suffer from chronic pain of an unexplained source.

✳ Have a lower incidence of depression, eating disorders and panic attacks.

According to researcher Olga Pollatos, better interoceptive awareness might imply better strategies for emotional and physiological regulation.[148] Pollatos believes that some of the chronic pain suffered by people with poor interoceptive awareness may be the result of misinterpreting body signals as indicating threat. For example, she speculates that perhaps the pain of social exclusion could be felt as physical pain.[149]

Interoceptive awareness may also mitigate compulsive risk-taking, as demonstrated in studies looking at behavior in betting games. Perhaps greater awareness of the body allows quicker reading of a "gut sense" that caution is needed.[150]

This research makes sense by analogy to the relationship between movement skill and body awareness. Just as we would expect people with better perception of body position to have better control over movement, we should also expect that people with better perception of their internal state have better regulation of physiology and related emotions.

Although questions remain about whether interoceptive awareness is trainable through practice, this is an interesting line of inquiry which may shed light on the value of practices devoted to attending to information from the body.

✳ Summary

Movement and emotion are related in surprising ways. Mind-body practices have for centuries emphasized the benefits of moving with precision and directing nonjudgmental attention to sensations from the body. Science has already clearly established the benefits of these practices, and is now starting to understand the mechanisms. One way or the other, we can be assured that learning to listen to the body is a path well worth traveling. In the next section, we'll discuss how to find some good pathways.

PART III

THE PRACTICE OF MOVING BETTER AND FEELING BETTER

CHAPTER 8

STRATEGIES TO MOVE BETTER AND FEEL BETTER

"Warning: Before beginning a program of physical inactivity, consult your doctor. Sedentary living is abnormal and dangerous to your health."
— Frank Forencich

IN THIS CHAPTER, I WILL DISCUSS the "brain-based" strategies to move better and feel better that are used in the movement lessons in the following chapter.

I am listing them here because all of them can be used in other contexts, such as athletic training, physical therapy, yoga, Pilates, weight training, corrective exercise, or manual therapy. Understanding their rationale will help you better understand why your current practice is working, or not working, or can be improved in some way. Not all of these strategies will be appropriate in every instance, but they are all options that may or may not be useful at certain times.

Some of these techniques are oriented toward finding novel ways to move that may improve biomechanics. Others are more about creating the mindset that facilitates learning and neuroplasticity. Others involve trying to change how the nervous system perceives threat associated with movement. They are listed below in no particular order.

Play

The lessons in this book are intended to be more in the nature of play than work, because play facilitates learning and neuroplasticity. Play is encouraged by:

* Including movements that are fun or rewarding for their own sake

* Avoiding boredom and routine

* Encouraging exploration and creativity

* Using novel movements

* Focusing attention on the process of the lesson as opposed to the objective or end goal

Play is particularly useful in the context of solo practice, without a coach, and without any strict time limits. Plus, it's fun and motivates you to show up for practice.

Experimentation

The play in the lessons in this book is not random, but structured. Many of the movements are sequenced with the intention of creating a series of controlled "experiments" in movement that change variables and compare outcomes. For example, movements of the pelvis can be done with and without related movements of the head to determine which way of moving feels easier. One important aspect of an experimental approach is that it recognizes the value in doing a movement the "wrong" way. This clarifies if there is benefit to doing the movement "right."

Offering options versus prescribing corrections

The lessons are more about offering and exploring the relative merits of different movement *options*, as opposed to diagnosing movement *dysfunctions* and prescribing *corrections*. There are several advantages to this approach.

First, it avoids pathologizing potentially useful movement patterns. If you believe moving in a particular way is wrong, this will increase a perceived threat related to that movement. For example, even though it might be a good idea for you to avoid excessive low back flexion during a forward bend, this does not mean you should develop an unreasonable fear of low back flexion or completely avoid this movement.

Second, thinking in terms of offering choices as opposed to prescribing corrections respects the individuality of different people, and the difficulty of determining what movements are "right" or "wrong" for their particular structure. In other words, what is right for one person might very well be wrong for another.

Third, framing new movement patterns as a choice will help ensure they are used in a way that is organic, authentic and sustainable as opposed to forced, unnatural and temporary. There is a big difference between standing tall in a way that feels natural and effortless versus stiff and awkward.

Most people will abandon a "correct" movement pattern if it doesn't feel natural, or cannot be maintained without conscious attention. But some people with a lot of willpower will persist in adopting the unnatural movement pattern for long enough that it becomes a pathological habit. A connection to authentic movement is lost.

In either case, the correction fails if the deep unconscious part of the nervous system is not convinced the new movement pattern is beneficial. The solution is to offer options and test how they work, rather than ordering corrections and assuming they will work. If the new movement option is truly an improvement over the previous one, then the nervous system will show some sign it likes them.

Focus of attention and intention

The health of the body maps depends on properly interpreting proprioceptive information from the body. Directing attention to that information helps ensure it doesn't get ignored.

Because the scope of focused attention is limited, it can be beneficial to shift it from one part of the body to another, so as much sensory information can be gathered and integrated as possible.

For example, consider the movement of rolling the pelvis forward while sitting in a chair. You could focus on sensations coming from the hip joints, the abdomen, the low back, and the contact of the sit bones with the chair. Similarly, the same movement can be performed with different intentions: increasing flexion in the hips, rolling the pelvis forward, lifting the chest up and forward, or expanding the belly forward and down.

Each different intention or focus of attention will create slightly different movements and perceptions of the movement. Some of these variations will feel more or less natural, efficient or painful than others. The shifting of attention allows you to map the movement from different perspectives, distinguish subtle differences in how the movement is executed, and ultimately choose the version of the movement that is most efficient and comfortable for you.

Further, paying attention to the effects of a particular movement in a distant joint can help educate the brain on mechanical patterns of work distribution, which are an important element of coordination. For example, if you notice how your head moves in response to movements of your pelvis, you will gain greater awareness of the functional connection between these two areas.

An internal focus of attention may be appropriate in a rehab context, where you are trying to break bad habits of movement and perception. An external focus is more appropriate in a performance context, where the goal is optimizing healthy patterns. For example, if you wanted to improve your throwing accuracy, most of your attention should be directed externally (e.g. whether you hit the target), as opposed to internally (what your scapula is doing as you throw). But if you are trying to break a bad habit of moving the shoulder that is causing pain, then you might need to direct attention to exactly how the scapula is moving to find different ways to move.

Finding a reference for correctness

The brain needs feedback to assess the correctness of a movement and make changes to improve it. If there is no objective external evidence of the correctness of a movement (such as a ball going into a basket or a teacher giving feedback), the evidence must come from interpreting self-generated sensory information.

For example, if you want to reduce excess tension in your shoulders, you need to be able to feel the difference between more and less tension! In these lessons, you will be asked to make subtle distinctions between the level of effort, comfort and smoothness of different ways to perform the same movement. The hopeful result is an increased awareness of subtle differences in movement quality that will promote motor learning.

Slow gentle movement

Moving slowly is an effective tool to help change perception, motor control, and threat associated with movement. Here are seven reasons to go slow!

1. Slow movement is required if you want to move with deliberate intention and focused attention. Fast movements begin and end before you have time to notice anything.

2. Slow movement increases the amount of time you have to process sensory information about body position during movement. If you wanted to create a detailed map of a city, at some point you would need to slow down enough to drive through all the side streets and alleys. If you only drove fast, your map would include only the location of the highways. Movement is in many ways the same. If you want to map all the movements of your shoulder joint and assess the relative comfort of the many different angles it can move, you will gain far more information by moving slowly.

3. Under the "Weber Fechner" rule, slow and gentle movement reduces the magnitude of the sensory stimuli associated with the movement, and therefore increases perception of differences in the magnitude and character of the stimuli. In simpler terms, it is easier to tell the difference between one and two pounds of pressure than it is to tell the difference between 100 and 101 pounds. In the context of movement, this means the slower and more gently you move, the easier it

is for you to know if you are using excess effort or tension to perform the movement.

4. Slow movement preferentially recruits motor units with fewer muscle fibers, which have better control of force output. Faster more powerful movements will recruit the larger motor units that are less precise. Thus, slow movement is an effective way to improve postural control, which should be provided by tonic slow twitch postural muscles, as opposed to phasic fast twitch prime mover muscles.

5. If you move quickly, your repertoire will be limited to "feedforward" movements that are well practiced or habitual. Slow movement is required if you want to move in novel or unpracticed ways. To use the skiing down the mountain analogy, if your priority is to get down the mountain as fast as possible, you will always select the deepest, most well-worn groove. It is only when you are content to go down the mountain slowly that you will find other tracks or pathways that have been neglected, but may in fact eventually become faster once they have been used for enough repetitions.

6. Moving slowly reduces the perceived threat associated with movement because it decreases mechanical forces to their minimum. Thus, slow movement is an important tool in a plan of graded exposure that can allow you to explore and try movements you may have neglected for years because they are perceived to be unsafe and involuntarily restricted.

Graded exposure

Graded exposure is the progressive introduction of threatening movements or other stimuli, in the right dosage and timing, which causes the nervous system to become *less* threatened by the movements. In other words, if you painlessly perform a movement that used to hurt, your nervous system will find that movement less threatening in the future. We can look at graded exposure as a plan for "threat inoculation." This is a very simple and important concept in understanding how movement can reduce pain.

If a child wanted to convince his overprotective mother that it was safe for him to play at the playground, he would first need to show her he can play without getting hurt. A good strategy would be to start slowly with the safest activities, and then progressively move to more dangerous ones, all the while showing her he is safe from injury or threat. Hopefully, Mom will chill out at some point. You can go through a similar process of graded exposure to show your nervous system that a particular movement is safe. If running three miles causes your nervous system to freak out, try running just one and see if that is acceptable. If so, slowly inch the mileage upward and monitor the response.

If you perform some movement without pain that normally hurts, your brain is likely to get very interested. It is "good news" that reduces threat. A major goal of any program for movement health should be to send as much "good news" to the nervous system as possible about the state of the body and its ability to withstand the stress of movement.

In the context of the lessons in this book, good news might come in the form of performing a movement that has been neglected for some time, perhaps due to previous injury. For example, if rotating the head to the left is normally painful, it may help to find some other way to rotate the head to the left which is not painful, such as moving very slowly, rolling the head on the floor, or having the head moved passively. One of the main strategies in these lessons is to find ways of moving that might normally be uncomfortable, but will feel good with novel modifications.

The benefits of graded exposure can be seen in the context of almost any exercise program that employs progressive overload. If you safely and comfortably perform a heavy deadlift, run many miles, move through a challenging range of motion at a joint, or move explosively with power, these are all forms of good news to the nervous system about the health of the body. (They also lead to favorable adaptations in the tissues!)

The simple formula for success is this: Move as much as you can without hurting yourself, wait for the body to adapt, and try to move a little more next time.

Novelty

Novel movements have several potential benefits. They get the brain's attention, which enables changes in perception, neuroplasticity, and sensory gating effects on nociception. They also encourage use of movement patterns that are non-habitual and may lead to new solutions to motor challenges.

Imagery

Imagining a movement activates the parts of the brain that perceive and control that movement. And it will probably not activate any pain neurotags associated with the movement. This helps break the potential connections between the pain and movement neurotags.

Functional relevance

The brain will not be interested in reorganizing the way it moves the body unless the new way of moving can help with the performance of important functions.

For example, your brain is not likely to care very much if it learns how to activate the serratus anterior better in an overhead reach. But it might be very interested in learning how to throw a ball without pain, or how to press more weight, or how to reach farther, or do whatever it is you want to do.

The movements used in these lessons are likely to be viewed by the brain as being relevant to the performance of functional tasks for several reasons. They are done in developmental positions that the brain recognizes as the environment in which it learned movement in the first place. The movements are usually presented in the context of some function, such as reaching, orienting the head to see the environment, or transitioning between two positions.

Developmental positions and movements

Developmental positions are used for the reasons stated in the chapter on development. They will:

* Encourage the use of fundamental movement patterns

* Reduce threat and stabilization demand

* Increase proprioceptive feedback through contact with the floor

    * Increase opportunities to use closed chain movements and fixed points for movement that are not available standing

Plus they are fun and relaxing. A quick formula for making up your own movement session based on developmental positions is:

1. Get into a developmental position such as crawling, sitting, squatting, supine, prone, etc.

2. Perform a developmental task such as reaching, orienting the head to see, or transitioning to another developmental position.

3. Move playfully, mindfully, comfortably, slowly and reversibly.

Constraints

The lessons often constrain certain movement or stabilization options to require the nervous system to start using different movement patterns that might currently be underutilized or neglected. This is often done by performing a movement while maintaining contact between two different body parts, such as placing a hand on the head, the knee, or the foot.

Another common constraint is to perform multisegmental movements while only using certain segments. For example, turn the trunk all the way to the right while letting the head also turn right, then try turning while keeping the head still. This constraint demands more movement in the thorax, and clarifies the relative contributions of different segments in turning. To use the team analogy, we improve the performance of the thorax by forcing it to perform while the neck is on the bench. After a little practice, the neck returns to the field and there is better teamwork. Put another way, practicing "differentiation" often results in better "integration."

Another key constraint is the requirement to move slowly, smoothly and with a minimum of ballistic assistance. This is to ensure that movement between positions is controlled at every point along the movement arc. One test for this control is the ability to reverse the movement smoothly at any point. Another test is when the movement is done at a constant speed, so it does not appear "ratcheted" or jerky.

Repetition

Repetition is an essential element of learning. Thus, getting your reps in is important, especially when trying to break a habit or establish a new one. Far fewer reps are required when the goal is to simply activate or recover an old pattern.

Avoiding pain

Contrary to the popular phrase "no pain, no gain," moving in the presence of pain and discomfort has several disadvantages.

1. There are many ways that pain can breed pain. Nociception can sensitize peripheral and spinal nociceptors, facilitate pain neurotags in the brain, and strengthen unwanted neural connections between pain and movement.

2. It is very hard to learn anything new about movement while in pain. Pain will catch the brain's attention and make it harder to focus on the sensory information coming from the movement. And pain makes movement that might be fun or playful turn into an unpleasant chore. Thus, the presence of pain creates a poor learning environment.

3. Pain leads to perception of threat, which may lead to undesirable protective mechanisms like increased stiffness, decreased flexibility, decreased strength, and altered coordination patterns. Thus, it can be very counterproductive to attempt to retrain motor control in a painful area.

One caveat: the instruction during these lessons to not move into pain should not be confused with the admonition to *never* move while in pain during the activities of everyday life. This can lead to sedentarism and excessive fear of movement that could increase perception of threat and pain.

Avoiding threat

Even in the absence of pain, the nervous system may perceive threat related to movement and take undesirable protective measures like creating excessive stiffness and muscle tension. These lessons include various methods to reduce threat associated with movement, including moving slowly, trying to make movements as comfortable as possible, and moving in developmental positions on the floor that require less stability and balance. Further, they direct attention to subtle indications of threat, such as holding the breath or excess muscle tension, particularly in the hands or face.

Avoiding fatigue

The lessons in this book should be done in a way that does not create any fatigue or exercise stress. Although exercise that causes fatigue is very beneficial in building the health of the body and brain, in some ways, it can interfere with motor learning. Moving while fatigued can impair the ability to focus attention on sensory feedback, discourage the use of novel movement patterns, and create threat that causes protective mechanisms. Although many classes in yoga, Pilates, or functional training strike a good balance between exercise stress and motor learning, the strategy employed in these lessons is to divide and conquer. Thus, if the movements cause any fatigue, frequent rests should be taken.

❄ Summary

If I had to quickly summarize all the above strategies to move better and feel better, I might offer the following:

Move playfully, experimentally and curiously, with full attention on what you are doing and what you are trying to accomplish.

Focus on movements that are the foundation for your movement health, and have a lot of carryover to many activities, as opposed to movements that are specific and don't have carryover.

Move as much as you can without injury, pain or excess threat, wait for the body to adapt, and then move more next time.

In the next chapter we will present some specific lessons that illustrate one way to implement this strategy.

CHAPTER 9

LESSONS IN BETTER MOVEMENT

"Make the impossible possible, the hard easy, and the easy elegant."
— Moshe Feldenkrais

"Strength that has effort in it is not what you need; you need the strength that is the result of ease."
— Ida Rolf

THIS CHAPTER SETS FORTH twenty-five lessons for improving your movement and perception. These represent ONE example of how the strategies listed in the preceding chapter can be applied. They are based on the Feldenkrais Method, which was developed to help people learn to move with greater efficiency, comfort and awareness. (For more information on the Feldenkrais Method, see http://www.bettermovement.org/the-feldenkrais-method/)

These lessons are especially appropriate for people who want to improve their movement, on their own, without a coach or equipment. They are potentially useful for people of almost any skill level, age or physical ability. Before getting started, here are some guidelines to observe while doing the lessons to ensure maximum benefit.

1. Never move into pain

Make sure you stay comfortable during the lesson and feel better after the lesson than when you started. If a particular movement causes pain, reduce the range of motion or the speed of the movement. You can also try imagining the movement. Or just skip it altogether and focus on movements away from the area of pain.

Fortunately, because the different body parts work as a team, you can change the way a painful area moves and feels by moving a non-painful area. For example, if your shoulder hurts, it is probably best not to start with a lesson about shoulder circles. Try a lesson directed at the spine and see if that helps.

2. Pay attention

The lessons describe a series of movements as well as places to direct attention. Focus of attention is just as important as the movement! However, the exact direction of attention isn't mandatory. The directions in the lessons are just suggestions. Think of your own variations or follow the sensations you find interesting. One way or the other, don't just go through the motions!

3. Rest

The lessons suggest various places where you should pause or rest. These are just suggestions. Pause or rest whenever you like, and certainly whenever you feel physically or mentally fatigued. Rest in any position you like, but resting on your back is best, because this provides the best opportunity to pay close attention to sensory information from the body. The first lesson called Body Scan provides a long list of things you can observe about the body as you lie on your back.

4. Develop a "feel" for good movement

While doing the movements, it is helpful to have some sense of what movements are to be preferred over others. One way to do this is to keep in mind some of the qualities of good movement discussed at the outset of the book: efficiency, relaxation, coordination, reversibility, balance, comfort, and a good distribution of effort.

But it may be even more helpful to develop an aesthetic appreciation for your movement quality. A picture is worth a thousand words. So, you can imagine moving in some way that you find pleasing, comfortable or graceful. For example you could picture:

* A cat stretching on the floor

* A baby rolling to the side

* A tai chi master shifting weight

* A dancer raising an arm

* The movement of a lion stalking prey

* The way you would walk on the beach during a relaxing vacation

You should also refine your internal sense of when a movement feels authentic, natural or "right." Good movement often has a quality of feeling effortless or involuntary when it is being controlled at a more subcortical or reflexive level, which is often a good sign.

5. Play and experiment with the lessons

Some lessons prescribe a choreographed series of movements, while others are more like templates that allow you to combine movements in different combinations. At the end of most lessons is a section called Variations. You should definitely explore the variations, but usually only after you have repeated the basic movements enough to see some improvements. Make up your own variations.

6. Which lesson?

Some of the lessons are more basic and fundamental, while others are more advanced and complex. The lessons are *roughly* organized to proceed from more fundamental to more complex. The breathing and long spine lessons are particularly foundational, and the squatting lesson is probably the most difficult. But you can do them in any order you choose.

While many of the lessons center around a movement in one part of the body, (e.g. the shoulders), each lesson involves coordinated activity from many joints. Thus, don't assume a lesson with the word "shoulder" in the title is the best way to address problems with your shoulder.

7. How much time to spend on the lessons?

The lessons do not prescribe a certain number of repetitions for each particular movement, or a specific time to complete a particular lesson. Some should take at least twenty minutes (not including variations) and some can be done in as little as five to ten minutes.

For any particular movement in a lesson, repeat it as often as you have the interest, focus and ability to pay close attention or improve it in some way. Even though some of the movements may feel simple and ordinary, approach them with the curiosity of someone who has never done them before — like an alien or a baby. This will help you notice sensations that you normally ignore.

8. Equipment

All you need to do these lessons is some comfortable floor space and time free of distraction. Some of the lessons involve sliding movements, and for these it is better to be on a floor that does not have excess friction. (In other words, a yoga mat won't work very well for some of these, but will be fine for others.)

Let's get started!

THE LESSONS

1. Body Scan

Purpose

To clarify "smudges" in the body maps and develop skill in focusing attention on subtle sensory information from the body. This is an effective way to reduce stress and pain all by itself.

This lesson is divided into sections. Spend at least a couple minutes on each section. You can do all the sections together as a standalone lesson. Or you can do small parts of the lesson as active rest during the pauses in the other lessons.

In some ways, this is a very difficult lesson in that it asks some questions about body sense that may seem extremely subtle to some people. It doesn't matter if you cannot find any clear answers to the questions. The benefit is more in the asking than the answering.

Imagery

Lie down on your back with your arms and legs extended. Spread the feet a comfortable distance apart. Relax and sink into the floor.

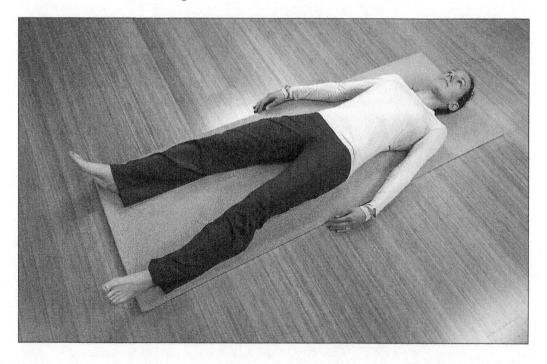

Even though there is no work to be done in this position, you may find that you continue to carry some degree of muscle tension. Find it and let it go.

Are you holding some parts of your body away from the floor, as if you're unwilling to let them "fall"?

Imagine what your body would do if someone pulled the plug on your nervous system, or you just died. Would your body move at all?

Contact

Notice your contact with the floor. Which parts of your body make contact and which do not?

Imagine you are lying in wet sand. If you stepped away, you would see an imprint showing how your weight was distributed on the ground. Some parts of your body would leave a deep imprint, some would barely make an impression, and some would make none at all. What would your imprint look like?

Here are some specific areas of focus to help you develop your body awareness.

Feet

Where do your feet point? Straight up toward the ceiling or out to the side?

Which foot points away from you more? Note the precise point where your right heel makes contact with the floor. Is it the same on the left?

Legs

Are the backs of your knees in contact with the floor? Which knee is bent more?

What part of your lower left leg touches the floor? How wide is the area of contact? What part of the upper left leg makes contact? Is this pattern the same on the right side?

Which leg *feels* longer to you? Which leg feels larger? On which side is it easier to sense the outline of your leg? For example, one leg may feel fuzzy or hard to locate in space, while the other comes very easily into your awareness. Build up your image of the legs as much as possible, as if you were constructing an internal model.

Pelvis

Where do you feel most of the pressure on your pelvis and sacrum? Is it equal on the right and left sides? Don't try to change anything, just notice how you are lying right now.

How well distributed is the weight throughout the pelvis? In other words, is every different part of the pelvis bearing an equal amount of weight, or do you feel there are certain small areas that have a lot of pressure and others that have almost none?

Where exactly do your legs meet the pelvis? Do you locate this area near the bony projections on the outside of the hip? Or closer to the groin? Which leg feels more functionally integrated into the torso, as if it has "roots" in the belly or spine?

Spine

Trace the line of your spine from the tip of the tailbone through to the top vertebra of the neck. Where is the top vertebra of the neck? Behind your throat? Behind your nose? Your eyes?

Try to imagine each vertebra one by one along the chain. Which segments are easier to locate in your mind's eye? Which ones are fuzzier?

How high and how long is the arch of your low back away from the floor? The arch in your neck? You can use your hands to explore either space to test your awareness.

Shoulders

Feel the contact of the shoulder blades with the floor. They are shaped like triangles. Does the triangle rest flat against the floor or does one end tip upward? Compare the contact of the right shoulder blade with the left. Which is more flat to the ground?

Arms

Note the contact of the upper arms with the floor. Which upper arm rests more fully into the floor?

What do you do with your hands? Are they palm down or palm up? Or in the middle? Do your fingers hold any tension? Which hand is curled more into a fist?

How well integrated are your arms into your torso? Where does your arm start? At the shoulder joint? Or closer to the middle where the clavicle meets the sternum?

Head

Where does your nose point? Directly toward the ceiling? Or angled a little forward or back? Or to the left or right? Are your facial muscles and jaw fully relaxed? Release any tension and note if this makes you feel any more comfortable or relaxed.

Breathing

As you breathe, where do you feel the most movement — the belly or the ribs? Does your spine change its contact with the floor as you breathe?

Midline and cardinal lines

Sense the midline of your body from the center of the forehead through the chin, through the sternum and pubic bone. How well are you able to imagine the continuity of this line?

Imagine the five cardinal lines of your body: the spine, two arms, and two legs. Which line *feels* longest? Which line *is* longest? Which line is easiest to draw, or jumps most quickly into your awareness? Which line is fuzziest?

As you imagine the lines of the body, what is your perspective on the body? In other words, do you imagine yourself looking from the right, left, straight above, or from where your eyes are right now?

2. Lengthening the Spine

Purpose

To improve perception of spinal position and the coordination of the deep local stabilizer muscles that align the vertebrae.

Movements

1. Assume your normal posture (the way you would stand without thinking about it) and assess your overall level of comfort and the position of your head, shoulders and chest. Place your feet hip-width apart and point the toes straight ahead. Equalize the weight on your feet so it falls just in front of the heels.

2. Visualize the length of your spine from the tailbone to the top of the neck.

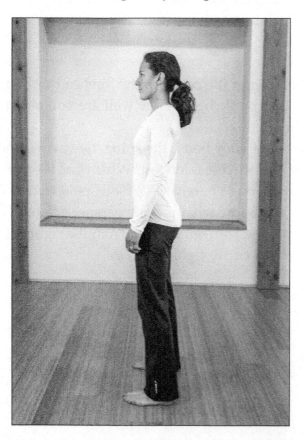 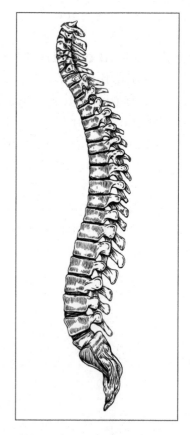

How deep in your body do you locate your spine? Do you visualize the back of the vertebrae — the tails that form visible bumps on the skin? Or the front — the circular bodies that lie deeper in the body? Try to visualize the line of the bodies of the vertebrae — the deep central axis around which the trunk is organized.

3. Lengthen your spine from the tailbone to the top of the neck. You can imagine that a string is pulling your head up from the crown of the head.

This is easier if you take your hand and pull some of your hair on the crown of your head upward.

4. Continue to lengthen the crown of the head up and now imagine a weight is attached to your tailbone and pulling it downward.

Imagine as the spine lengthens, the space between each vertebrae grows, as if the discs were inflating with air.

5. Continue to lengthen and find the segments of the spine that are more difficult to visualize.

Move your attention systematically from each segment of the neck, thorax and low back to find the "blind spots." Focus your attention on these areas so you can imagine there is some lengthening occurring there.

6. Relax into your normal posture for a minute. What changed? Did you grow shorter? Why?

7. Lengthen the spine again, imagining you want to touch the crown of your head to a ceiling that is slightly overhead.

As you do so, what movements, if any, do you notice? Can you feel the muscles around your back or trunk working differently?

8. As you lengthen, does your head tilt back? Make sure the back of the neck stays long, so the chin stays down and slightly tucked.

9. As you lengthen, do the ribs in the front raise or become more prominent? Visualize lengthening the spine while keeping the lower ribs in the front down, as if you wanted to make them disappear. Make sure you're not holding your breath.

10. Relax and reassess your posture. Is it taller, better aligned? Easier to maintain?

11. Walk around a little and see if you can maintain a tall spine as you walk. Could you walk around like this all the time? What would it be like to walk into your place of work or a social event in this posture?

Variations and Progressions

Try the same exercise in different configurations:

* The arms straight out in front of you, to the sides, and overhead

* The trunk rotated right and left

* On hand and knees

* Tall-kneeling, half-kneeling

* Bent at the waist so the trunk is forty-five degrees to the ground

It is beneficial to maintain a long spine position while doing any (almost) form of resistance exercise, including front and side planks, pushups, farmer's walks, pullups, presses, rows, squats, deadlifts, and lunges. In each case, the resistance will tend to pull you out of alignment. Maintaining a long spine in the presence of these forces is probably the best and easiest way to train functional core stability. Try one of these exercises and notice that even a small degree of lengthening of your spine against resistance will make the exercise feel *very* different.

3. Breathing

Purpose

Breathing involves the coordinated action of almost every muscle in the trunk, from the pelvic floor to the neck. The key movements are the rise and fall of the diaphragm and the expansion and contraction of the ribs.

These same movements contribute to trunk mobility and stability. In particular, the downward movement of the diaphragm creates intra-abdominal pressure, which is an essential aspect of spinal stability. This lesson is a way to explore and recover ways of moving the diaphragm and ribs that you may have habitually neglected. This can affect the coordination and strength of the entire trunk.

Seesaw breathing

1. Lie on your back with your feet standing on the floor and the knees pointed toward the ceiling. Observe your breathing for a few rounds and note where you feel movements associated with breathing and where you do not.

2. Take a large breath into your belly so it expands like a balloon. Hold your breath and move the "ball of air" from your belly to your chest, so the chest expands maximally and the belly sucks inward as much as possible, like a vacuum.

3. Continue to hold your breath and move the ball of air back and forth from the belly to the chest, expanding one as you contract the other. Now exhale and breathe normally and relax. (Don't hold your breath too long!)

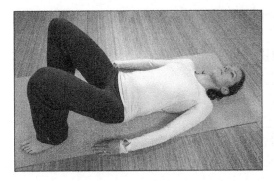
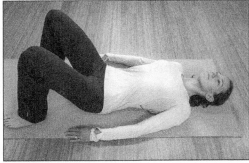

4. When you are ready, repeat this same "seesaw" movement enough times so you can gain awareness in regard to the following.

Alignment of the spine

5. As you blow the ball of air back and forth, do you feel the back alternately arch and round? Try to keep the spine in the same alignment as you move the air, so your contact with the floor does not change very much. This will test your ability to differentiate movements of the diaphragm and ribs from movements of the vertebrae.

Even expansion of belly and chest

6. As you blow the ball of air up and down, can you feel that some parts of your belly and chest inflate more easily than others? Is it easier to breathe into the right or left side of the belly? Which part of the chest expands easier?

7. Try to equalize the inflation in all areas. Make sure the belly is expanding to the side and not just toward the ceiling. Place your thumbs on your side waist just below the lower ribs and your fingers on the lowest outer portion of the abdomen to make sure you are able to inflate these areas that are often neglected. Think of expanding like a balloon in all 360 degrees.

Selective expansion of the belly and chest

8. Can you direct the ball of air so the right side of the belly and chest inflates more than the left? Try the reverse to see which is easier.

9. Can you move the ball of air diagonally — from the right belly to the left chest? Which diagonal is easier? Make sure you are moving the ball of air with a minimum of movement in the spine.

10. Can you fill your belly with air until your body literally starts floating to the ceiling? Just kidding.

Reverse breathing

11. Here is a different way to breathe. Inhale while sucking the belly inward and expanding the chest outward. Then exhale while depressing the chest

and inflating the belly. Again, make sure your spine remains in neutral as you breathe. Try for even expansion in all directions.

Breathing with constant belly expansion

12. Inhale and exhale while always keeping the belly expanded in all directions equally, especially to the sides and near the groin. Use your fingers to find the areas that are hard to keep inflated as you exhale. Can you feel any tension coming into your neck? If so, try raising your head with a pillow to see if this becomes easier.

 ## Variations and Progressions

You can try any of these three breathing techniques (seesaw, reverse and constant IAP) in different positions which will create very different patterns of muscle activation.

* **Prone or child's pose**: This will facilitate expansion of the ribs in the back.

* **Side-lying**: Lie on your right or left side to facilitate breathing on the up side.

* **Supine twist**: Lie on your back with the arms extended to the sides and the legs tilted right or left. This will open the ribs on the opposite side of the legs.

* **Quadruped**: Compare the ease of breathing into different areas in various degrees of spinal flexion and extension.

* **Any difficult position**: If you are struggling with any of the lessons in this book, a yoga pose, or any position along a particular movement arc, such as the bottom of a squat, assume that position and then perform some of the breathing movements. Ensuring that you can breathe in a particular position is a way to "own" it.

4. Flexion/Extension Patterns in Quadruped

Purpose

To improve mobility and distribution of motion of the spine into flexion and extension and to integrate movements at the shoulder, ribs, diaphragm and hips.

Movements

1. Come to your hands and knees. Make sure the hands are under the shoulders and the knees are under the hips. If your wrists are uncomfortable bearing weight at this angle, you can use your fists or find a wedge that will reduce the angle of your wrists with the floor.

> *Visualize the length of your spine from the tailbone through the top of the neck and out the crown of the head. Imagine that you have a long tail in the back like a dog. Lengthen the spine.*

2. Move the middle of your back toward the ceiling and then lower it toward the floor so you are alternately arching and rounding the back. This movement is sometimes called cat/cow or cat/camel.

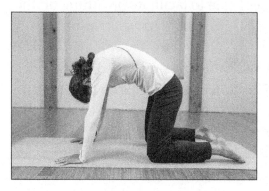 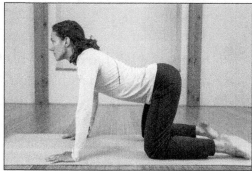

3. Repeat the movement enough times, and slowly enough, for you to sense which segments of the spine move independently and which parts feel stuck together like a block.

4. Pause.

5. Repeat the movement and focus on the movement of the pelvis. As you round your back, tuck your tail under as if you wanted to see it. Then as you arch your back, lift your tail behind you as if you were pointing it toward the ceiling.

> *Where does your head want to look as the tail moves up? As the tail moves down?*

6. Pause.

7. Continue the same movement, and as you tuck the tail under, look down to the tail. As you lift the tail to the ceiling, look up to the horizon.

> *Don't hyperextend the neck as you are looking to the horizon. Keep the back of the neck long, and imagine lengthening the crown of the head to the ceiling.*

8. Pause.

9. Begin arching and rounding again and notice the movements of your navel. As you arch downward, inhale into your belly to expand it toward the floor like a balloon. Move so the navel "leads" the downward movement of the front of your trunk.

10. As you round the back upward, exhale to bring the navel as far as possible toward the ceiling. Continue to move back and forth for a few rounds, synchronizing your breath with your movement and expanding the range of motion of the navel in either direction.

11. Pause.

12. Continue arching and rounding your back and bring your attention to the movements of the sternum. Try to lower the sternum as close to the ground as possible, and raise it as high as possible to the ceiling.

> *How do the movements of the shoulder blades cooperate with the movements of the sternum? Can you feel them sliding closer and farther from the spine?*

13. As the sternum moves downward, allow the shoulder blades to move closer to the spine and down the back. As the sternum moves up, allow them to spread wide.

14. How far are your shoulders from your ears as you arch and round? Try to keep a maximum comfortable distance between your shoulders and your ears.

15. Pause.

16. Continue the movement and assess the quality of contact between your hands and the floor. Which one makes a more solid contact? Do you press more with the inside or outside of the palm? Equalize the pressure on both sides of the palm and point the middle finger forward. Spread the fingers. How does your hand contact affect the quality of your movement?

17. Pause.

18. Repeat the original movement without focusing on any area in particular. Has the quality and ease of the movement changed? Is there better distribution of motion?

Variations and Progressions

You can practice this basic pattern of flexion and extension in many different positions. This will create constraints that require more movement in particular areas. Play around with the following options to challenge your mobility and coordination:

* Instead of resting on the hands, rest on the elbows and forearms with palms down

* Asymmetrical: one side rests on the hand, the other on the elbow/forearm

* Pelvis on the heels, with either hands or forearms on the floor

* Staggered stance: Left elbow and knee farther from each other than right elbow and knee (and vice versa)

* One knee crossed behind the other

5. Coordinating the Flexors

Purpose

To coordinate the flexors on the front side of the body, including the deep neck flexors. This may improve their function as stabilizers of the spine, help prevent excess extension, and/or reduce tone in the extensors of the low back.

Movements

1. Lie down your back.

> *Feel the space under your low back. Is the space big enough to place a deck of cards?*

2. Lift your head to look at your feet. Repeat the movement a few times so you can sense what muscles work to create the movement, the effort required to lift the head, and how high the head lifts easily. Does this strain the neck muscles?

3. Bring your feet to standing so the knees point to the ceiling. Lift the right foot so you can get a hold of your right knee with your left hand.

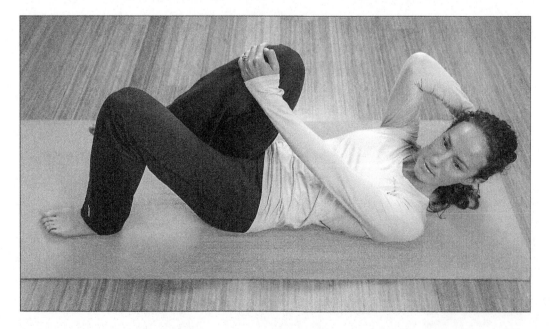

4. Place your right hand behind your head so you can feel the weight of your head in your palm.

5. Use the right hand to help lift the head and bring the elbow and knee together. Don't try to touch them together, just move a comfortable distance and then repeat.

> *Feel how your ribs and sternum move down to allow the head to lift. Exhale as you lift the head and inhale as you lower so you move in sync with your breathing. Try to make the movement as effortless as possible.*

6. Pause.

7. Now switch the left hand over to holding the left knee and put the right foot back on the floor. Then use the right hand to lift the head and bring the right elbow toward the left knee. You are now flexing at a slightly different angle. Feel how your ribs and sternum move down and slightly left as you lift the head.

> *What is the most comfortable place for the head to look as the right elbow goes to the left knee? Allow your head to turn off to the left as it comes up and see if that makes the movement easier.*

8. Pause.

9. Switch your hands so the right hand is holding the left knee and the left hand is behind the head. From this position, bring the left elbow and left knee together. Repeat many times.

> *Sense how the contact of your back with the floor changes as you lift and lower the head. The upper parts peel away from the floor while the middle parts press more into the floor. Which parts of your back provide the most support to lift the head and knees? Do you roll more to the left side or the right side of your back? Pay special attention to the part of your back under the low ribs and try to press this into the ground as the head lifts.*

10. Pause.

11. Let go of the left knee and let the left foot come to the floor, then get a hold of the right knee with the right hand. Then bring the left elbow and right knee together and repeat many times.

> *As the head lifts, think about bringing the crown of the head as close to the ceiling as possible, as if you were trying to get a view of the horizon. How does this change the movement?*

> *Again, use as little effort as possible. If you are shaking, holding your breath or breathing hard, reduce range of motion and increase rest periods between reps.*

12. Pause and rest with the legs extended.

> *How high is the arch under the low back now? How long?*

13. Interlock your hands and place them behind your head. Then lift both feet from the floor so your knees come over your belly. Exhale and use the hands to lift the head to bring the elbows and knees together. Then inhale and allow the head to come back down and repeat several times.

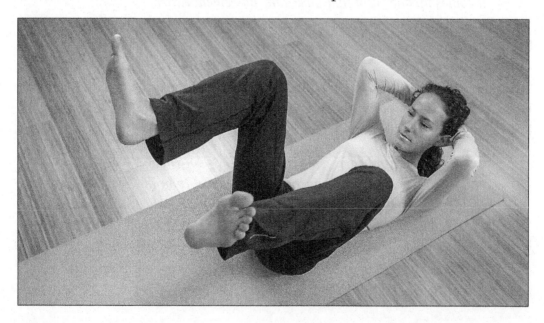

Feel how the upper chest peels away from the ground as you exhale. Think of bringing the lower ribs down so you make them disappear. Press more into the ground directly under the low ribs.

As you lift the head, think about lengthening the back of the neck so the chin does not poke forward but instead tucks slightly. Push the crown of the head to the ceiling.

14. Pause.

15. Return to the same movement. Can you lift the head while keeping the arch under the low back? Or is it easier to flatten the low back into the floor as the head lifts?

16. Start to direct the left knee to the right elbow, then the right knee to the left elbow, and play with different combinations to find which angles of flexion are easier, which ones are more difficult. Roll around on your low back to feel all the points on the low back press into the floor to support you.

17. Let your leg go long, and take a rest.

18. Lift the head a few more times and look at the feet. Has this movement become any easier? Does the head feel lighter?

19. Stand and walk around and notice if your chest feels more open. Paradoxically, it is sometimes easier to open the front side of the body when it gains more skill in closing.

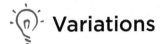 **Variations** ———————————————————

Try similar movements of lifting the head with the following variations:

* With one or both legs extended

* Lifting the head while pulling the hair on the crown away from you to encourage the neck to lengthen

* Using one or two hands to guide the sternum into the floor and down to the pubic bone to encourage the chest to fold

6. Coordinating the Extensors

Purpose

To coordinate the activity of the many muscles which extend the spine, hips and neck.

Movements

1. Lie down on your stomach. Place your hands palm down, one on top of the other, with the elbows out to the side. Then rest your chin on the hands.

2. Look to the wall in front of you and raise your eyes and head to look up the wall and then to the ceiling above you. Allow your chest to peel away from the floor to look farther above you. Repeat this several times.

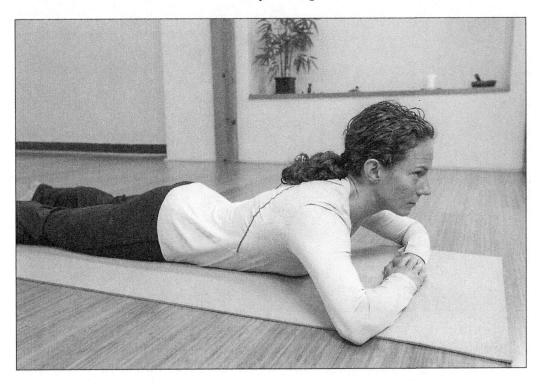

How much effort is required to lift, and how far can you look with comfort? Do you feel pinching or excess effort in the low back? In the neck?

3. Place the right hand over the left and rest your left cheek on top of the right hand so you are looking to the right elbow. Get comfortable.

4. Imagine your cheek is glued to the right hand. Lift and lower the right elbow and right hand, and your head that is glued to the right hand. Try to keep your right forearm parallel to the ground as you lift and lower. Repeat many times.

> *As you lift and lower, sense the change in the contact of your chest with the floor. Can you feel the chest press into the floor more? Do you roll a little bit to one side? Find the areas of the chest that provide the best support for lifting.*

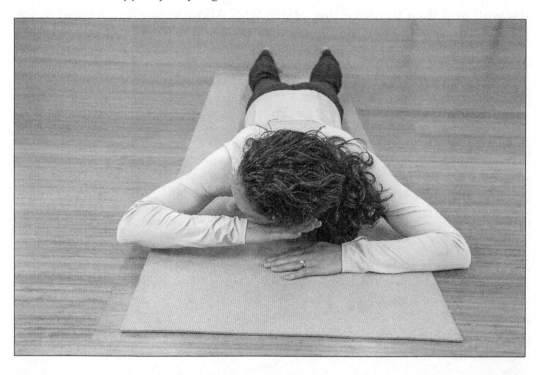

5. Turn your face to the left and switch over your hands so the right cheek is resting on top of the left hand. Then repeat the same moves by lifting and lowering the head and left forearm.

> *As you did before, find the part of the chest that provides the best support for lifting.*

Do your legs respond to the movement of the arm and head? If you had to lift one knee and foot from the floor as the left arm lifts, would it be the left or the right leg?

6. Pause.

7. Lift and lower the right foot and knee from the floor just an inch or two and repeat this several times.

Feel the muscles in the back of the leg and the low back work to help lift the foot. As the foot lifts, do your head and arm get lighter against the floor?

8. The next time you lift the right foot from the floor, lift the left arm and head from the floor at the same time, and then lower it to the ground at the same time. Repeat many times.

Sense how the movement of one limb makes the other lighter. Feel the part of your chest or belly that presses more into the floor to support the lifting of the opposite side limbs.

9. Pause.

10. Switch your hands over so the right hand is on top of the left and rest your head on the left cheek so you can look to the right elbow. Lift and lower the right arm and head a few times and sense which one of your legs becomes lighter on the floor. Don't assume it is the left leg! Find your habitual pattern.

11. Pause.

12. Lift and lower the left foot a few times until you can feel that the lifting of the left foot invites the right arm and head to lift. Then lift the left leg and right arm at the same time so you can feel how these movements counterbalance one another.

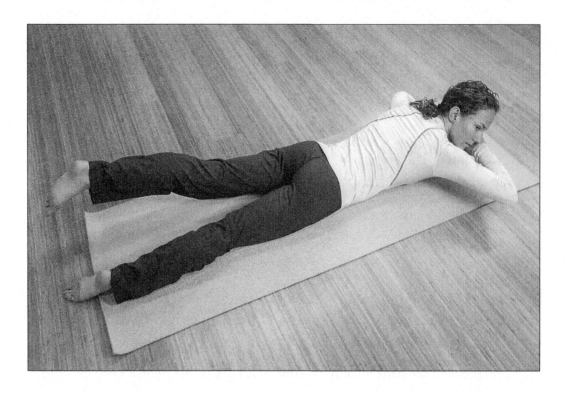

13. Pause.

14. Place your forehead down on top of your folded hands and then lift the hands and elbows and head away from the floor so the forearms are parallel to the floor. Lift and lower several times, each time changing the point of support. Move from the chest, to the belly, to the pubic bone.

> *Which point of support allows you to lift highest?*
>
> *As you lift, what do the legs do? Try allowing them to lift and also try keeping them on the ground.*

15. If you like, try sliding your head and forearms to the left and the right a few times in the air after lifting them to a comfortable height. Feel how your chest moves to create the movement.

16. Pause.

17. Return to the movement we did at the beginning of the lesson. Keep your hands on the floor and lift your head and eyes to look to the ceiling, allowing your chest to peel away from the floor. Have you expanded your comfortable range of motion? Are you lifting with less effort?

18. Come to standing, walk around a little and see if you have a greater awareness of the musculature on the backside of your body. Is your chest more lifted?

19. If the back muscles feel like they are holding too much tension, you can relax them by doing some of the movements from Lesson 5 on Coordinating the Flexors.

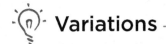 **Variations** ———————————

Here are some variations:

* Make small circles with the lifted foot

* Lift the foot with the knee bent and the lower leg vertical

* After lifting the head and arm, slide it right and left as if it were hovering over the ground

* Turn the head to face the hand that is down, and then lift the elbow and hand that is in the opposite direction of the arm you're lifting. Does this still activate the opposite side leg?

7. Coordinating the Side Flexors

Purpose

To coordinate the muscle chains on the sides of the body, including the hip abductors, the quadratus lumborum, the obliques, the intercostals, and the side neck flexors.

Movements

1. Lie down on your right side. Draw your knees up so the hips and knees are comfortably bent and the knees and feet are stacked. Make sure you are really lying on your right *side*, and your trunk is not rolled to the front or back.

2. Extend the right arm long overhead so it forms a continuous line with your spine and your head rests on top of the right arm. If that is not comfortable, you can have the right arm extended out in front of you.

3. Wrap the left arm over the top of your head so the left hand can get a hold of the right ear.

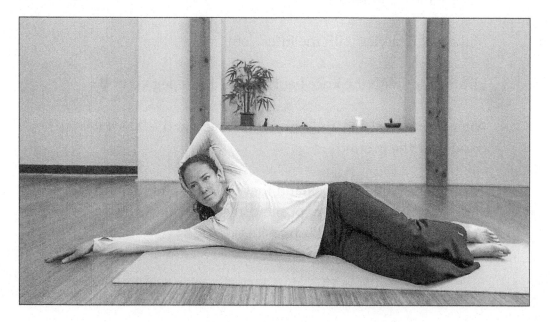

4. From this position, lift the head as if you were trying to see the horizon. Move just far enough to find a comfortable range of motion, then repeat many times.

> Try to make this a pure side-bending movement. You can imagine your body is sandwiched between two walls and you don't want to touch them as you move.

> How heavy is the head and how far does it lift with ease?

5. Lower the head and rest. You can bring the left arm down in front of you.

6. Lift the left foot away from the right *while keeping the left knee on top of the right*. Lower and repeat many times.

> As the foot moves, does the crest of the pelvis move to the ribs? (i.e. the left side waist shortens). You can allow that to happen in order to lift the foot higher.

7. Rest.

8. Extend the left leg long so it forms a continuous line with the spine from your head to your foot. Keep the left leg long and lift the left foot from the floor as high as comfortable and lower it many times.

> Can you feel the right side waist press into the floor as the left side waist shortens? Does your head get lighter on the floor or feel invited to lift along with the foot?

9. Pause.

10. Wrap your left hand around your head as you did before. Now lift the head and the long left leg at the same time. Lower them together and repeat many times.

> Does lifting the foot make the head lighter?

11. Rest and re-stack the left knee on top of the right. Now lift the head a few times with the left hand and see if the movement is becoming easier.

12. Roll onto your stomach.

13. Interlock your hands and place your forehead in the hands. Keep the forehead glued to the hands, and slide your hands over to the left in an arc and then back to the middle and repeat this many times.

> *Feel the right side ribs open up like an accordion as the left side ribs close. Try to reduce friction as you slide. How far do you go comfortably?*

14. Pause with your head in the middle.

15. Slide the left leg over to the left as far as it will go and leave it there. Then slide the head and hands left again.

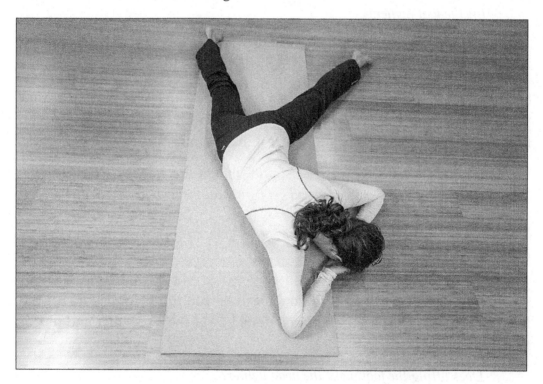

Does the position of the left leg allow you to slide the head farther to the left? Slide it back and compare your quality and quantity of movement with the left leg in different positions.

16. Roll onto your back.

17. Interlace your fingers and allow your head to rest in the palms. Then, as you did on your stomach, glue the head to the hands and slide them in an arc to the left, sending the left elbow in the direction of the left hip. Make sure the face stays oriented directly to the ceiling so the head does not roll.

18. After you've done this a few times, start sliding the head to the left *at the same time* you slide the left foot to the left. Alternate between sliding the head with and without the foot to compare differences.

19. Come to standing and walk around a little and feel the differences between the two sides. Which side feels longer? Can you feel how the muscles on the left side support you as the left leg swings forward? If you notice a significant difference between the sides, lie down and repeat some of the same movements on the other side.

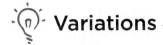 ## Variations

Quadruped sidebending

Come to your hands and knees. Bring your feet and knees together. Pivot on the knees so the feet swing left and right.

As you do that, turn your head to look at the feet. Feel how this movement alternately bends one side and then the other. This is kind of like a side bending version of the cat/cow exercise.

As you did in that lesson, try to distribute the work of side bending evenly through the spine and integrate movements of the pelvis and scapula with the spine. Play with speeding the movement so it is light and quick. Crawl around to see if you can feel how one side shortens and lengthens as you move.

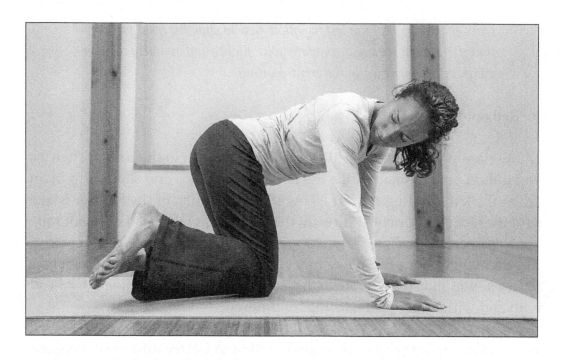

Sidebending in standing

Reach the left arm all the way to the ceiling, as if you are really trying to reach something above you. Feel how the whole left side of your body lengthens. Which foot bears more weight as you reach with the left hand? Let your weight shift fully to the left foot, so you lengthen the whole left side, pressing the left heel into the floor and the left hand into the sky.

Then perform the same movement on the right side, allowing the left hip to rise and the left side to shorten.

Then alternate from side to side, reaching one hand then the other, while shifting weight to the same-side foot. Which side lengthens easier? Which Michael Jackson video comes to mind? (Hint: Beat It.)

8. Improving Rotation

Purpose

To improve coordinated rotation of the pelvis, spine and shoulders.

Movements

1. Lie down on your back and draw your knees up so the feet are standing on the floor and the knees point to the ceiling.

> *Sense the contact of your pelvis with the floor. Which side of the pelvis bears more weight? Which side of your low back feels farther from the floor? Which shoulder blade is flatter to the floor?*

2. Gently tilt your knees from side to side toward the floor so you feel your body twisting from the pelvis through to the shoulders.

> *Note the comfortable range of motion and the quality of the movement through the spine and ribs. Where do you feel the motion is stiff or restricted?*

3. Cross your right knee over your left knee so there is no space between the thighs. You will be standing on the left foot as the right foot dangles in the air.

4. Tilt your knees over to the right in the direction of the floor, return them to vertical, and repeat this movement many times.

> *Find the first place along the movement arc where you feel a restriction. Don't move past that place of resistance — wait for that place to move farther right.*

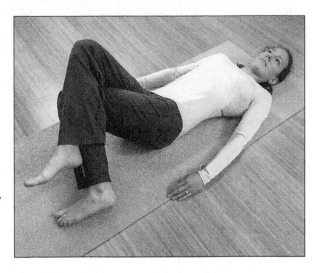

5. Pause with your knees in neutral.

6. Bring the palms of your hands together and point them to the ceiling so your arms form a triangle. Make sure the elbows are completely straight.

7. Maintain the exact position of the triangle with the hands together and the elbows fully extended, and tilt your triangle over to the left. That means your right shoulder will lift from the floor to roll your chest a little to the left.

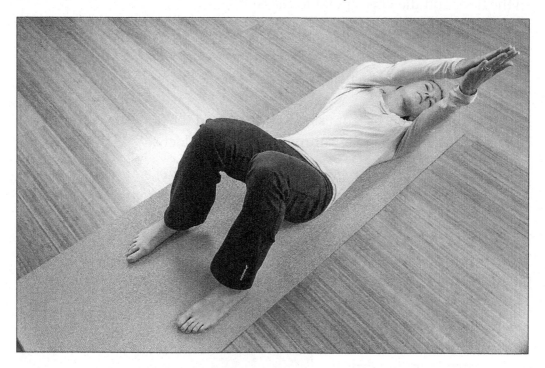

Make sure you're not cheating by bending the left elbow. Feel the muscles that work to roll you to the left. You are actively performing the same rotation that was done passively by tilting the knees.

8. Pause and bring your arms down to your sides.

9. Tilt your legs over to the right again and see if this movement is becoming any clearer. Feel the ribs on the left side open to allow the twist.

Does your head respond to the movement of the pelvis? Allow the chin to move down to the chest as the knees tilt right.

10. The next time your legs tilt right, let them hang out a comfortable distance from the floor.

11. Keep the knees in place, interlace your hands and place them behind your head. Use the hands to lift the head so your nose moves directly to the left hip. Repeat several times.

Does the movement of the head affect the position of the knees? The activation of the stomach muscles will tend to pull the knees a little back to the center. You may find that each time you lower the head, you're able to lower the knees farther to the right.

12. Pause and let your legs extend. Which side of the pelvis rests more into the floor? Which shoulder blade?

13. Cross your left knee over the right and tilt them to the left side a few times. How is this side different than the right?

14. Move your legs far enough to the left so you can feel the right shoulder being pulled away from the floor. When you reach this position, keep your knees in place, and then actively press the back of the right shoulder to the floor a few times so you can feel the muscles on the back side of your body working to increase the twist.

15. Bring your knees back to the middle and pause.

16. Tilt your knees to the left again and let them hang a comfortable distance from the floor. Now, as you did in Lesson 3, Breathing, inhale a ball of air into your belly, hold your breath, and move the ball of air back and forth from the belly to the chest.

Which parts of the belly are easier to inflate? As the belly expands and contracts, can you feel the knees moving back and forth?

17. Bring both feet to standing and rest for a minute. Feel where your breathing happens in the belly. Roll your head from side to side a few times to release any tension in the neck.

18. Extend both arms straight out to the sides. As you did before, tilt your knees from side to side and compare the quality of this movement to the start of the lesson. Feel how the belly expands to allow the lower back to arch from the floor; how the ribs open on the opposite side; how the chin moves to and from the sternum.

19. Let the legs fall from side to side very lazily and comfortably a few more times to release any tension throughout your whole trunk and spine.

20. When you're ready, come to standing and sense the rotation of the hips, spine, ribs and shoulders as you walk.

9. Rolling like a Barrel

Purpose

To reduce excess muscle tension while at the same activating deep spinal stabilizers in a relaxing and pleasurable rolling movement.

Movements

1. Lie down on your back and bring your knees into the air so you can hold both knees with both hands. The arms should be passive and responsive like ropes.

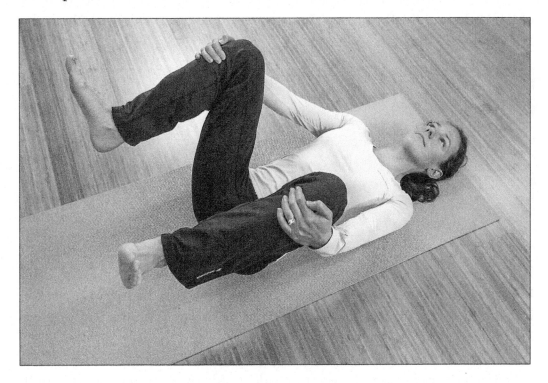

2. Use the hands to bring the knees far apart and then touch them together. You can think of them opening and closing like a book.

3. Open and close the book several times until you can find the maximum comfortable distance for the knees to fall open. Then leave them there with the hands on the knees.

4. Feel the contact of your back with the floor. Is your low back arched from the floor or flat? Roll the pelvis back and forth on the ground so you can explore different ways for the pelvis and low back to contact the floor. Then find a comfortable neutral position.

5. Feel the roundness of the cylinder of your rib cage. Breathe into your belly, especially in the sides, and all the way down into the groin. Let your back spread wide against the floor.

6. Using your left hand, pull the left knee down and to the left until the left elbow and left knee touch the floor. Allow the right knee, head, and the rest of the body to roll left until you are resting on your left side with the right knee on top of the left.

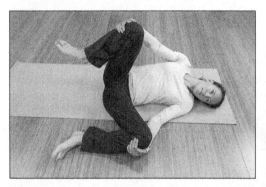 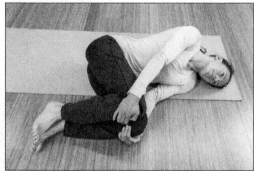

7. Pause for a minute in this position, then use the right hand to pull the right knee away from the left until it pulls the left knee and the rest of the body into a roll onto your back and then to your right side with the left knee on top of the right.

8. Very gently and smoothly roll from side to side by using the hands to pull the knees in the direction you want to go.

> *You can think of the knees as a steering wheel for the hands to move the body back and forth. Notice that it takes just the lightest pull on the knee to initiate rolling to either side.*

9. As you roll to your side, make sure not to crash into the ground. Find a way to roll that does not require momentum. You can ensure that your movement is completely controlled and balanced at all times by preserving your ability to reverse your movement in the opposite direction.

10. Keep breathing into all corners of your abdominal cylinder, so the belly expands in all directions like a barrel. Allow your back and ribs to be round and responsive to the floor, so you are able to find support and balance from any part of the trunk.

11. Notice the speed and rhythm of the rolling of your head. Roll it at a constant slow speed from side to side. Make it pleasurable and hypnotic. Allow the head to either lead or follow the movement of the knees, but always find a pleasant rhythm.

12. Continue to roll and release tension throughout the body, even as you find a sense of deep support and activation from the core of the body.

⟨ƞ⟩ Variations

Try similar rolling movements with the knees and feet in similar positions, but with the hands *not* touching the knees. Raise the hands and feet in the air and roll from side to side as if you were holding an imaginary gym ball between them. Keep the hips, knees and ankles all at ninety degrees. This will require more stability and control.

10. Rolling from the Back to the Side

Purpose

A fun way to reduce global tension, coordinate deep chains of trunk stability, and integrate the arms and legs with the trunk.

Note: Because this lesson involves sliding movements, it should be done on a surface without excessive friction.

Movements

1. Lie down on your back with the legs extended and your arms on the floor above your head.

> *How far do the arms comfortably extend? How high is the arch in your low back? Do you breathe more in the belly or the chest?*

2. Slide the backs of your hands to the left while sliding both feet to the left until you feel yourself rolling into a ball on your left side with the knees close to the elbows.

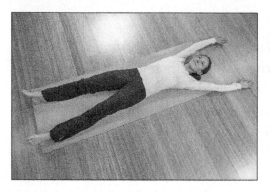 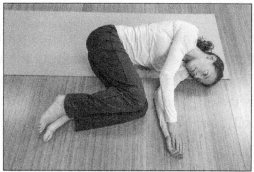

3. Now reverse the movement by sliding your hands and feet back where they came from until you are lying in the starting position — on your back with the arms and legs extended.

4. Move back and forth between these two positions many times by sweeping the hands and feet in long, lazy arcs on the floor. As you do that, direct your attention as follows:

* Make sure the hands and feet always maintain contact with the floor, so you are sliding them, not lifting.

* Initiate rolling through the reaching and sliding of the arms, while letting the pelvis and legs roll passively. Think of your lower body as a rag doll. (This is easiest when you are rolling from the side to the back.)

* As you roll to your side, which knee bends and slides left first? If you go very slowly and let the legs respond to the roll of the pelvis, you will feel the left leg bend and slide left first, and the right leg will lag behind. Then on return, the right leg will extend first and then the left leg.

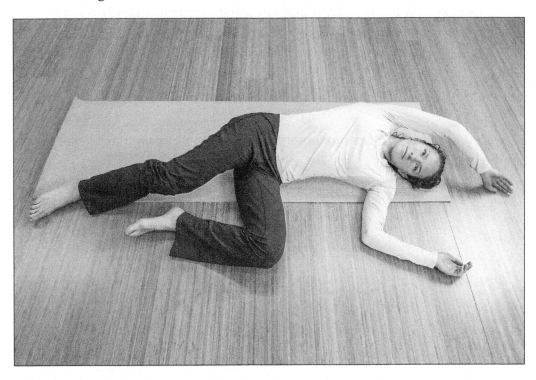

5. Pause and rest on your back.

6. Extend the arms overhead again and roll to the right. On return, continue rolling to the left and then roll from side to side.

> *Notice your body is opening and closing as you roll. Exaggerate this motion by moving into a tight fetal ball on your side and fully lengthening the arms and legs on your back.*

7. Continue to roll but move as slowly as possible. Take fifteen seconds to complete a cycle, moving at a constant speed with a minimum of tension. This will ensure you are always in control of the movement, even as your point of support is constantly changing. Are you balanced and comfortable at every point?

8. Now speed the movement up as fast as possible for a few cycles.

> *Does moving quickly clarify anything about the coordination between the core and the extremities? Feel how the core pulls the arms and legs inward.*

9. Slow down again and see if the quality of your movement has changed at all.

10. Can you use a similar movement onto roll to your stomach? No? Then try the next lesson.

11. Rolling from the Side to the Stomach

Purpose

Like the previous lesson, this one seeks to reduce global tension in the trunk, increase coordination of the oblique muscle chains, and integrate the arms and legs with movements of the trunk. This lesson is also best done on a surface without much friction.

Movements

1. Lie on your stomach with your legs a comfortable distance apart and your arms on the floor above your head. Roll your pelvis a little to the left so the right hip lifts from the floor. Allow your right knee to bend and your right elbow to bend so they can slide a little bit closer to each other. Repeat this motion several times.

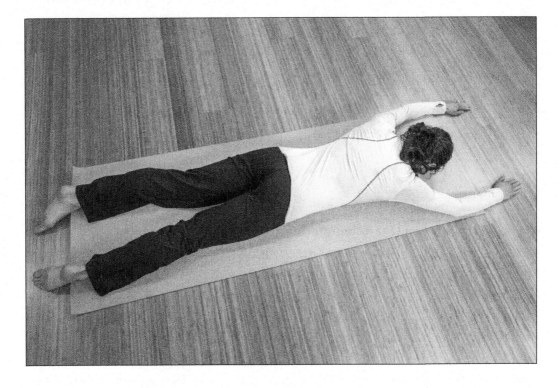

2. Pause.

3. The next time you roll onto the left side of your pelvis, allow your left arm to slide underneath your head so the left elbow can move toward the left knee and you can rest on your side with the arms and legs bent.

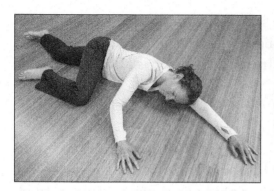 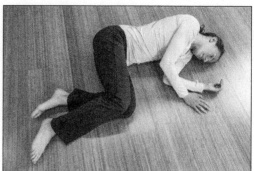

4. Reverse the movement by extending both your arms back overhead and straightening the legs so you are on your stomach. Repeat this several times.

> *Notice the sequencing — the right elbow and knee move together before the left elbow and knee move together. On the way back to the stomach, the order is reversed.*

5. Next time you are on your stomach, try making the same movement to roll onto your right side.

> *Each time you roll, find the timing and coordination to make this movement light and easy.*

6. The next time you roll to your stomach, keep going so you roll to your left side, and then keep rolling from side to side through the stomach. As before, you can change speeds to reveal different ways to coordinate this movement.

7. The next time you're on either one of your sides, try to incorporate the movements from the previous lesson by rolling onto your back and then onto the next side, and then onto your stomach, and then keep going (depending on how much floor space you have). Play around with these opening and closing movements, finding how you can roll across the floor simply by opening and closing the arms and legs.

8. You can perform this quickly to activate your core, or very slowly and gently to reduce muscular tension in a hypnotic and pleasurable way.

9. Have fun with this and make sure to explore different ways to sequence it — the movement can be "led" with different parts of the body — the right hand, the left hand, the foot, the pelvis, the head, etc.

10. You can also try to make sure the movement is always reversible at any point, so you are always balanced and adaptable.

12a. Releasing the Neck Part One

Purpose

To relieve excess tension in the neck, and break neural associations between pain and movement of the neck.

Movements

1. Lie down on your back. Place the palm of your left hand on your forehead with the elbow out to the side.

2. Imagine the hand and forearm are a wooden board and the head is a ball. Move the hand and forearm so the head rolls from side to side.

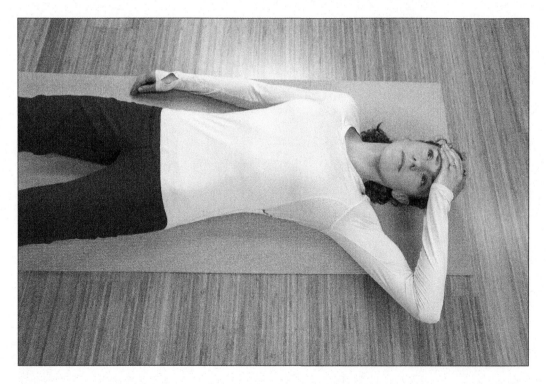

3. Keep the muscles in the neck completely passive — the head turns only from the power of the arm, and without any muscle activity in the neck at all. It's harder than it sounds! Soften your jaw, your eyes, and the corners of your mouth.

4. Try the same movement with the right hand. Again, try to keep the neck as passive as possible so the hand turns the head, not the neck muscles.

> *The absence of muscle activity in the neck reduces compression of the vertebrae, which may reduce nociception that is normally associated with rotation. This allows the brain to break associations between pain and movement, and reduce perception of threat related to movement.*

5. Put your hands down by your sides and rest.

6. Now, without the use of the hands, slowly roll your head from side to side. Use the rolling to sense the contour of your skull.

> *Is your head perfectly round, or does it have flat areas followed by ridged areas? Is it the same shape on the left as the right?*
>
> *As you roll your head to the left, can you feel the weight of your jaw falling to the left? If not, what holds it in place? Let your jaw, your cheeks, your tongue, your eyeballs respond to the changing relationship of gravity, and fall just a little bit from side to side as your head rolls.*

7. Start progressively reducing the distance you're rolling your head from side to side until you are approaching the middle point. Stop in the middle and rest.

8. When you're ready, come to standing, walk around, and slowly turn your head from side to side, to see whether you feel less tension in the neck and more freedom of motion.

12b. Releasing the Neck Part Two

Purpose

To activate the deep neck flexors and reduce excess tension in the neck.

Movements

1. Lie on your stomach and put your hands near your head. Rest on your forehead.

2. Move from your forehead to resting on your chin as if you are looking in front of you. Then move your head to look toward your navel. Try to peel the chest away from the floor to help you see as far down to your belly as possible. Move back and forth between these two positions, expanding your comfortable range of motion each time.

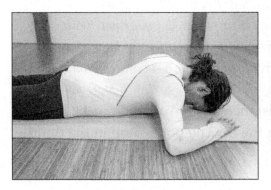 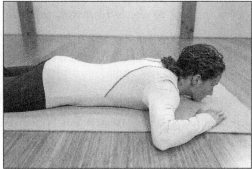

3. Pause and rest with your forehead on the floor.

4. Put your hands in a pushup position. Push into the ground with your left hand so you roll across the forehead until your head has rolled to face the left hand. Then push with the right hand so you roll back to the neutral position and then over to look at the right hand. Then use the hands to roll the head back and forth. Make sure the chin tucks a little so the nose doesn't bump on the floor. But otherwise keep the neck muscles relatively passive so the hands do the work. Repeat until you feel tension melting away from your neck.

5. Pause with the forehead in the middle.

6. Rest with your forehead on the ground, interlock your fingers, and place them behind your head. Lift your elbows away from the ground a few times so they are even with the hands. Feel the muscles between the shoulder blades working to help you lift the elbows. Try to minimize the downward pressure of the hands against the head.

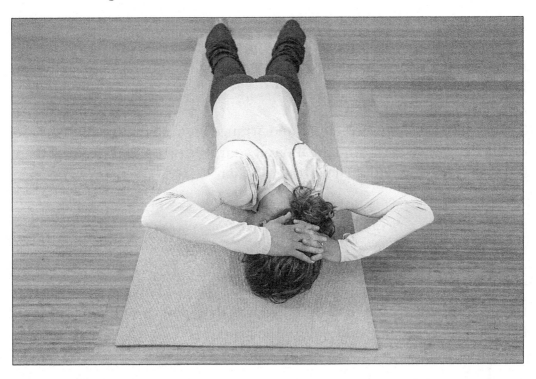

7. Keep the elbows in the air and then gently roll your head from right to left with the hands. Again, as before, try to move the neck passively, with the arms rolling the head side to side like a ball under a board.

8. Rest

9. Come to standing and notice the position and comfort of your head over your shoulders.

13a. Shoulder Rotation Part One

Purpose

To coordinate rotation of the arm with movements of the scapula, trunk, neck and pelvis. The movements in this lesson are also a good way to safely mobilize the nerves running to the arm.

Movements

1. Lie on your back with your feet standing on the floor and the knees pointed to the ceiling. Extend your arms out from the shoulders so they form a straight line out to the side.

2. Form soft fists with your hands and arrange them so they rest pinky side down. Keep the elbows straight and roll your fists up on the floor, and then roll them back down to their starting position.

> *Feel the rotation in the shoulder that allows the fists to roll. Take note of how far they can roll up comfortably. Can you roll them until the palm faces directly to the floor?*

3. Pause with your arms and fists in the starting position. Check to ensure the arms are straight out from the shoulders, the elbows are straight, and the fists are resting on the pinky side of the hand.

4. Again roll the fists upward on the floor, *but this time also lift your pelvis* into the air by pressing with your feet. This will allow you to roll the fists farther upward. Reverse the movement and repeat many times.

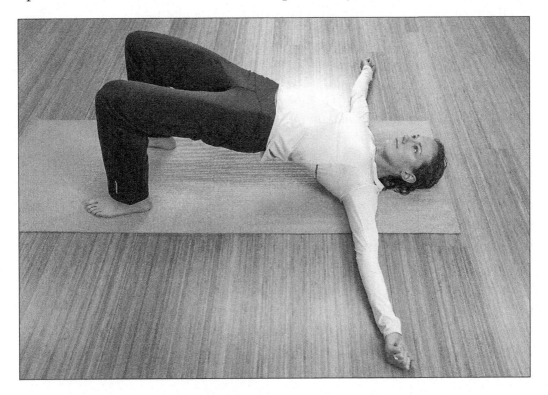

The higher you lift the pelvis, the farther you can roll the fists upward. Can you lift the pelvis until you are bearing weight under the two prominent vertebrae at the base of the neck?

5. Pause and rest.

6. Lift the pelvis again and roll the hands as far upward as possible, *then pin the fists in position on the floor,* and then lower the pelvis. When you cannot lower farther, lift the pelvis again and try to roll the hands farther up. Then pin them to the new position and lower the pelvis again.

> *As you lower the pelvis, let the vertebrae return to the floor one at a time, like links in a chain.*

> *Can you completely flatten your spine to the floor while leaving the fists rolled up to their maximum?*

7. Pause.

8. Now keep the pelvis on the ground and simply roll the fists upward and see if you have expanded your comfortable range of motion or if this motion is becoming smoother and more integrated.

9. Pause. Check to see that your arms are directly out to the sides, you are resting on the pinky side of the fists, and the elbows are straight.

10. Now roll the fists *downward* and note your comfortable range of motion on the right and the left.

> *Can you feel that your shoulders pull away from the floor to allow the fists to roll downward? Allow that to happen. Is your range of motion the same on the right as the left?*

11. Pause.

12. Roll the fists down again but this time also lift the head to look down at the toes. This will allow you to roll the fists farther down. Then roll the fists back as the head lowers and repeat this motion several times.

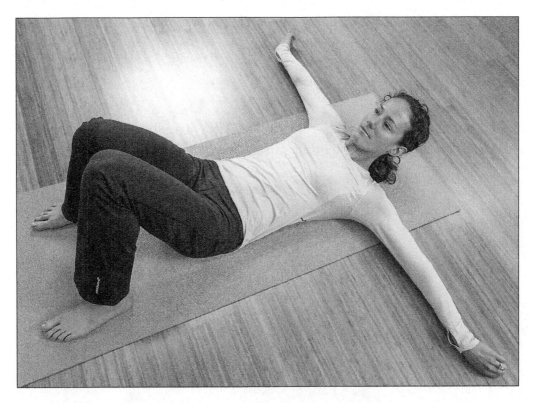

Feel how these movements work together — the lifting of the head, the rolling forward of the shoulders, the collapsing of the chest, the downward movement of the ribs, and the rolling of the fists.

13. Pause.

14. Roll the fists downward and lift the head until you reach a comfortable maximum distance of rolling, *then leave your fists in place* and start lowering the head to the ground. Feel the movements in the clavicles that need to occur to allow the spine to flatten against the floor.

15. Pause.

16. Now roll the fists up and down and note your comfortable range of motion.

> *Can you feel the activation of the muscles in the scapula? The movements of the scapula over the rib cage?*

17. Pause.

18. Roll one fist up as the other rolls down. Allow the shoulder rolling up to press into the floor while the other raises from the floor.

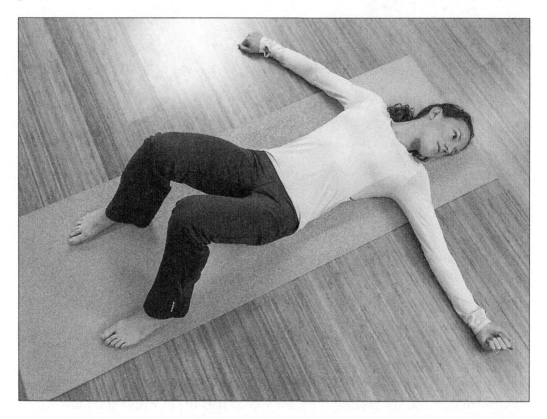

> *Can you feel your head being invited to turn by the movement of the shoulders? If you had to turn to look at either fist, would it be the fist rolling up or down?*

19. Continue to roll and try looking to the hand that is rolling up. Repeat many times so you can sense whether that feels natural, as if the shoulder movements are pushing the head from side to side.

20. Now try turning your head to the hand rolling *down* so the neck differentiates from the rotation of the shoulders.

21. Pause.

22. When you are ready, come to standing and feel the position of the shoulders on the chest. Walk and sense how the movements of the arms integrate with the trunk.

13b. Shoulder Rotation Part Two

Purpose

This lesson builds on the first, coordinating rotation of the arm with movements of the scapula, trunk, neck and pelvis.

Movements

1. Sit cross legged on the floor. Extend your arms straight out to the sides from the shoulder so they form a straight line parallel to the floor. Make fists with the hands and actively lengthen the arms outward.

2. Keeping the arms straight and the elbows extended, slowly rotate from the shoulders so the fists roll up. Return to neutral and repeat many times. Make sure the hands are always at shoulder height. (It is easy to cheat by allowing the hands to move down.)

Where does your head want to go? What does the sternum do?

3. Extend the arms again, and this time roll the fists up while looking to the ceiling. Allow the chest to expand as the hands roll up. Feel the shoulder blades move together toward the spine.

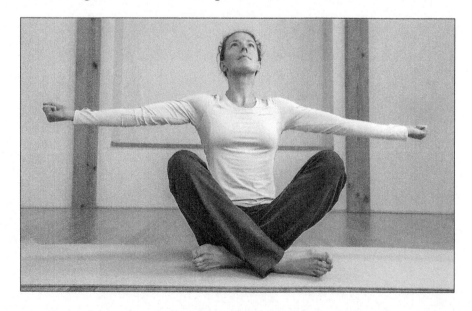

4. Pause.

5. Extend your arms again and roll the fists down. This time look down and allow your chest to slump. Notice that slumping allows you to roll the fists farther.

> *Exhale as the chest collapses. Allow the pelvis to roll back. Feel the shoulder blades widen on the back.*

6. Pause and rest.

7. Now put the two movements together. Roll the hands down and look down, then roll the hands up and look up. Let your eyes lead the movement and synchronize your breath. Make sure to include your pelvis in the movement.

8. Pause.

9. Now can you do the opposite? As the fists roll up, look down and allow the chest to collapse. Then as the fists roll down, look up and expand the chest.

> *This will be harder to do! Go very slowly and deliberately until the movement becomes easier.*

10. Pause.

11. Return to rolling the fists down while looking down, and rolling the fists up while looking up, and see if this motion is becoming any smoother, and you are coordinating more parts of yourself in the movement.

12. Pause.

13. Come to a kneeling position so you are standing on your knees and your feet are behind you. Extend your arms out to the sides and make fists.

14. Roll one fist down while the other rolls up. Turn your head to the fist that is turning up.

> *Feel how the turning of the shoulders is like the wringing of a towel. Does your chest turn to allow the movement? Can you feel your weight shifting from one knee to the other?*

15. Pause.

16. Perform the same movement except turn your head to look to the hand that is turning down.

> *Is this easier or harder than looking to the hand that turns up? Alternate to find out.*

17. Pause.

18. Stand your right foot on the ground in front of you while keeping the left knee on the ground under the left hip. Extend your arms straight out from the shoulders, make soft fists, and turn your body so your right arm is in line with the right thigh and the left arm is pointing behind you.

19. Begin wringing your arms again by turning one fist up and the other down. Look to the hand that is turning up.

> *Can you feel yourself leaning in the direction you look?*

20. As you look to the hand that is turning up, push that hand out away from you as if you were fencing. Make sure the hands stay at shoulder height, and feel how the rolling, turning and lunging all fit together into one integrated movement.

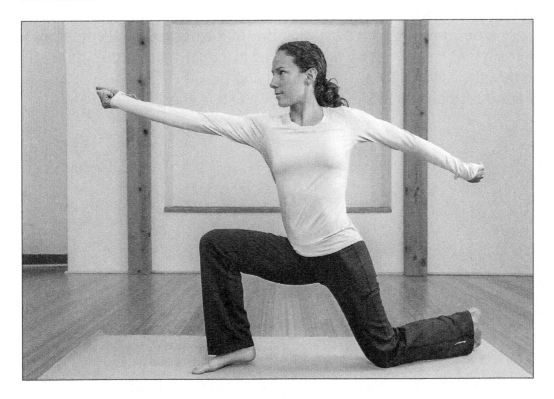

21. Reverse the movement so you lunge in the direction of the hand that is turning *down*. Then return to the more natural movement.

22. Switch your feet and try this on the other side. On which side are you a better fencer?

Variations

There are many ways to play with this movement. You can try leaning away from the direction you look.

You can also play with the sequencing of the movements. For example, you can start to turn one fist down and let that rotation help turn your neck to the other side, which turns the chest and the other shoulder up. As if a wave of rotation was moving from one fist to the other.

14. Shoulder Circles

Purpose

To mobilize the shoulder into a full range of motion while integrating movements of the ribs, spine and pelvis.

Movements

1. Lie on your left side with your hips and knees comfortably bent and both arms straight out in front of you. Make sure the elbows are straight and your right palm is resting on top of the left. You may want a pillow or rolled towel under your head for comfort.

2. Slide the right hand out in front of the left as if reaching for something on the floor a few inches away. Then slide it back, keeping the elbow straight. Make sure the right hand *slides* — no muscle effort is wasted in lifting the right hand to move it. Repeat the movement many times.

> *Is your right knee sliding forward over the left? Is your head rolling?*
> *You can allow your whole body to cooperate to let you reach farther.*

3. Pause.

4. Next time the right hand has slid past the left, start to slowly sweep it on the floor in an arc upwards. Go very slowly and curiously, sliding up and down, as if you were a baby exploring the floor with your hand. Watch the hand with your eyes and allow your head and trunk to roll as necessary. Imagine you are very curious about the texture of the floor.

5. Slide the hand up and down but work your way progressively upward. Make as wide an arc as comfortable, allowing the elbow to bend as necessary as the hand goes overhead.

6. Rest the hand on the floor when it is directly over the head, in line with the spine.

7. Now keep the left leg bent but straighten the right leg so it forms a continuous line with the spine and the right arm.

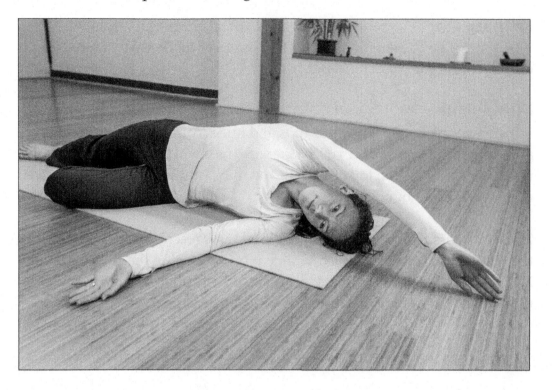

8. Feel the right inner heel on the floor and slide it *away* from you just a little bit.

> *This is a very small range of motion. If you are having trouble sliding the foot away, try sliding it toward you first and then away.*

> *As you slide the right heel closer and farther, can you feel the right hand change its contact with the floor?*

9. Next time you slide the right heel away from you, slide the right hand farther away from the head, so the whole right side of your body lengthens.

> *Feel how the left side shortens and the right side waist expands toward the ceiling.*

10. Roll to your back and take a rest.

Can you sense a difference between your right and left sides? Which side feels longer?

11. Return to your left side with the knees bent and stacked. Position the right hand directly overhead and in line with your spine.

12. Slide the hand behind the head until the hand naturally wants to turn from the front to the back. Sweep the hand back and forth across this transition point so you can feel the precise place where the hand wants to turn. Allow your head and whole trunk to roll in response to the movement of the hand.

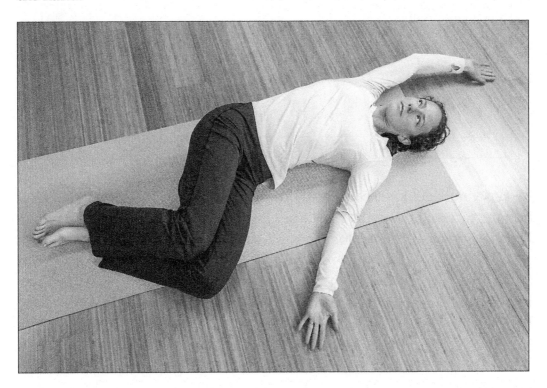

Move back and forth several times between these two positions so you can feel how the right side ribs and armpit needs to open to allow the right arm to lengthen and move down to the floor.

13. Now continue to arc the right hand around until it is straight across from the left arm. Make sure you allow the back of your right shoulder to come all the way to the floor so there is no strain in the shoulder joint.

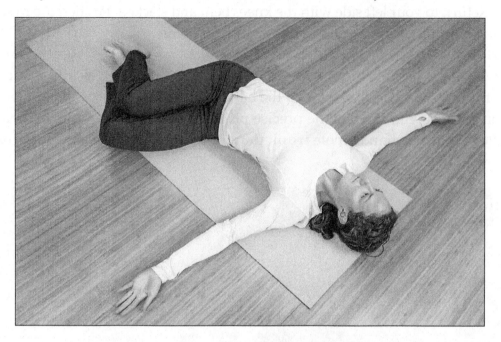

14. Has your right knee come away from the left knee? If so, leave the right arm in place and move the right knee just a little bit in the direction of the left a few times. Feel how this increases the twist in the spine.

15. Now let the right knee be free and continue to move the right hand down in a circle across and over your right hip until it is resting on top of the left-hand again.

16. Then repeat the whole circle several times, going very slowly, carefully and curiously.

> *Notice the connection between the arm and the body, and all the muscles that radiate at different angles to the ribs, the spine and even the pelvis. Feel how each angle of the arm will engage a different line of pull, and cause different compensatory movements of the trunk and pelvis. Work very slowly and patiently to equalize the tension in*

each angle so the movement is smooth, integrated, comfortable and pleasurable through each angle of the arc.

17. When you are ready, come to standing and walk around a little so you can discern the difference between your right and left side. As you swing the arms and walk, which arm feels more integrated with the trunk and the movement of the hips and the legs?

If you notice a significant difference, return to the floor and perform the same lesson on the opposite side. (If not, why bother?)

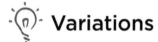 **Variations**

You can perform similar movements while standing near a wall. (You will need a lot of wall space.) To mobilize the right shoulder, stand with your right heel, right hip and right shoulder against the wall and take the right hand through a wide arc overhead, to behind you, to directly out front and then overhead again.

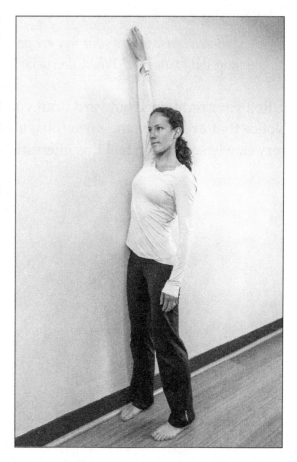

15. Primal Hip Flexion

Purpose

To improve hip flexion through a primal pattern that is seen in babies and reptiles. This pattern combines hip flexion with external rotation and abduction which helps centrate the hip joint. It may also preferentially activate the psoas over the other hip flexors (TFL, rectus femoris and adductors), which are not as well suited for centrating the hip.

Note: Because this lesson involves sliding movements, it is best to use a surface that does not have excess friction.

Movements

1. Lie down on your back.

> *Can you sense where your feet are pointing? Straight to the ceiling or more out to the side? Where does your heel make contact with the floor?*

2. Roll your right knee outward until you feel the right knee begin to bend. Notice that as soon as the knee rolls, it begins to bend. Roll several times very slowly so you can feel this interesting relationship.

3. Roll the knee farther until you can rest on the outside of the right foot. Then slide the right foot upward in the direction of the right sit bone. Then reverse until the right leg is extended. Repeat this movement many times very slowly and carefully so you can feel the interesting relationship between the rolling of the knee, the bending of the knee, and the sliding of the foot.

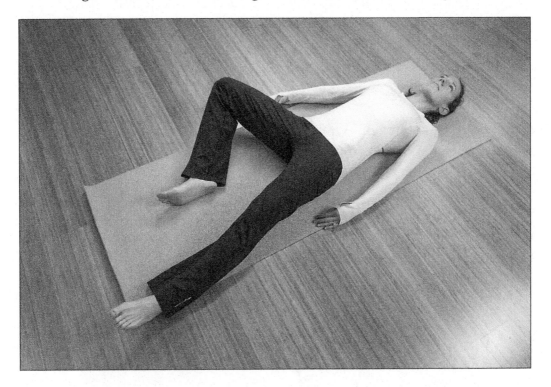

How high does the foot easily slide? For most people, this will be about the height of the opposite knee.

As you slide the foot up and down, let it fall out to the side so you can feel the muscles on the inside of the right thigh releasing.

4. Rest with both legs extended and compare the contact of your right foot to your left. Which toes point farther to the side?

5. Make a similar movement with the left leg, rolling the knee until it bends and allows the foot to slide upward.

Imagine a frog leg. How easily do the muscles on the inner thigh release?

6. After several repetitions, leave the left foot across from the right knee. Notice that you are resting along the edge of the left foot. Leave the left knee hanging to the side, and rock along the edge of the left foot, so the pinkie toes lift from the floor, and then the heel.

> *Imagine you are rolling on the edge of the foot like it's the rail of a rocking chair. As you do that, can you feel subtle movements in the hip joint?*

7. Extend your left leg and rest. Note the position of feet and the contact of the heels.

8. Roll onto your stomach. Arrange your arms so the hands are somewhere near your head and turn your head to the right. Spread your feet a comfortable width.

9. Roll your pelvis to the left a little bit so the right side of the pelvis lifts from the floor. As you do this, notice the right knee is invited to bend. Allow it to bend and slide the right foot and knee upward.

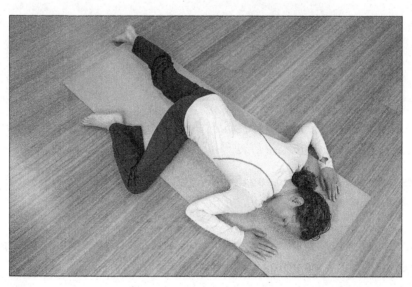

10. Do this many times very carefully so you can feel the sequence — the pelvis rolls, the right knee bends, and the inside of the right foot rolls to the floor and slides upward.

11. Turn your head to the other side and practice the same movement. Except this time, try placing your left hand in a pushup position so you can use the left hand to roll yourself a little bit more to the right to allow the left knee to come up. Once this becomes familiar, see if you can reproduce the ease of the movement without the assistance of the left hand.

12. Next time the left knee is drawn up near the waist, leave it there. Then roll your pelvis back to the left, so the left knee slides away from you, straight out to the side. Slide the knee back and repeat several times.

> *Notice how sliding the knee will stretch the muscles of the left groin. How close to the floor can you lower the left side of your pelvis as you slide the knee out to the side?*

13. Return to the movement of sliding the knee up and down and see if this becoming easier.

14. Roll to your back again and rest. Note the positions of the feet. Do they point more to the outside now?

15. Come to standing and walk around. As you flex the hip to bring the leg forward, can you feel an echo of the frog-leg movement?

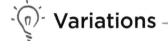 **Variations** ————————————————

Here are some variations on the same theme:

* As you lie on your back and slide the foot upward, does your pelvis change its contact with the floor by rolling slightly toward the sliding knee? Does your back arch away from the floor? Can you slide the foot while keeping the pelvis and low back stable?

* Slide one foot up as the other slides down. See if you can find a rhythm.

✻ Put one foot in the "up" position and slide the other foot up and down. Does this make it easier to stabilize the low back?

✻ Slide both feet up and down at the same time. Does your back arch away from the floor? Can you do it while keeping your back in neutral?

✻ Try rolling one knee *inward* until you can make a similar sliding motion upward, this time on the *inside* of the foot.

✻ On your stomach, put your hands in a pushup position and then slide one leg up and then the other. As one leg comes up, use your hands to help you lift and turn the head over or under the shoulder to see the leg coming up. Do you feel like a lizard?

16. Improving Control of the Hip in Deep Flexion

Purpose

To improve internal rotation of the hip and coordination of the hip in the deep flexion position that is required in a squat. This is a position that most people habitually avoid. **Note: This lesson might not be appropriate for someone with low back pain that is aggravated by low back flexion.**

Movements

1. Come to a sitting position with the soles of the feet together.

2. Lean on your left hand behind you and get a hold of your right foot by grabbing along the outside of the foot. The thumb should be together with the fingers, the palm on top, the fingers and thumb reaching to the bottom.

3. Use the right hand to lift the right foot to the ceiling and lower it to the floor and repeat this many times.

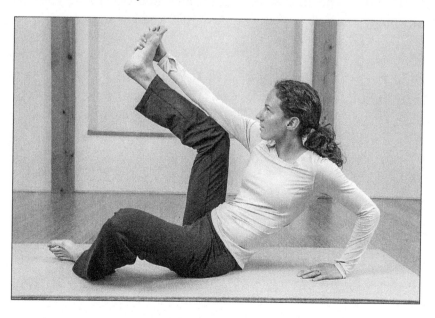

How heavy is the leg? How high does it lift with ease? Don't push through resistance to go higher, wait for the point of resistance to move

higher. If you don't have the flexibility to lift the foot, try holding it from a different place — the ankle or a pant leg. Or use a strap.

4. Release the right hand from the right foot and rest in sitting.

5. Get a hold of the left foot with the left hand in the same manner and begin lifting and lowering the left foot. Lean onto your right hand, so you can recline back.

Is this leg lighter or heavier? Let the left arm be like a rope, and allow it to lengthen as the foot lifts.

*Experiment with leaning back onto the right **forearm** instead of the hand. Which allows you to the lift the foot higher?*

6. Pause, roll onto your back and stand your feet on the floor.

7. Cross the right foot onto the left thigh so you can get a hold of the right foot with the right hand in the same manner as before. Place your left hand under your head.

8. Begin to lift the right foot to the ceiling with the right hand *while at the same time* using the left hand to lift the head. Repeat many times.

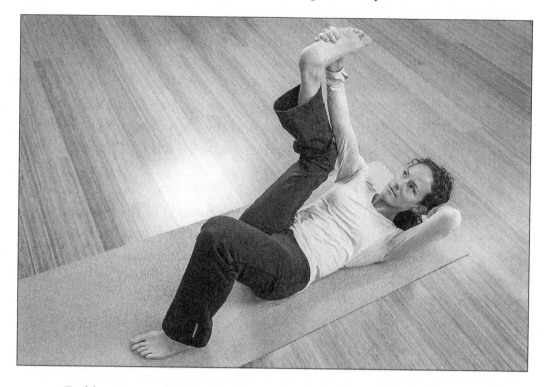

Feel how your whole body folds to allow the foot to come up. Let the foot be lighter each time you lift by reducing the tension in the leg. Lower the foot to the thigh and the head to the ground each time.

9. Let go of the right foot, place it on the floor and take a rest.

10. Cross the left foot onto the right thigh and get a hold of the left foot with the left hand, place the right hand behind the head, and repeat these movements on this side.

> *Notice how the pelvis rolls to the head to allow the foot to lift. Push the right foot into the floor for support. Feel how the left shoulder lifts from the floor to allow the arm to reach.*

11. The next time you lift your left foot into the air, *pass the left knee to the inside of the left elbow* so you can lower the sole of the left foot to the floor to the left of your body.

12. Then lift the foot and pass the knee to the outside of the elbow so you can lower the foot to the top of the right thigh. Go back and forth between these two positions, lifting and lowering the foot and passing the knee to the inside and outside of the left elbow. Feel what needs to happen in your hip, chest and shoulder to allow this movement.

13. Rest on your back for a minute and make sure your low back is not feeling any strain.

14. Return to a sitting position with the soles of the feet together.

15. Get a hold of the right foot as you did before and begin lifting and lowering the foot. Make sure the knee remains to the *outside* of the right elbow.

16. Next time you lift the right foot, allow the right knee to pass to the *inside* of the right elbow, and then lower the foot to the ground so the inside of the knee, lower leg and foot rest on the ground.

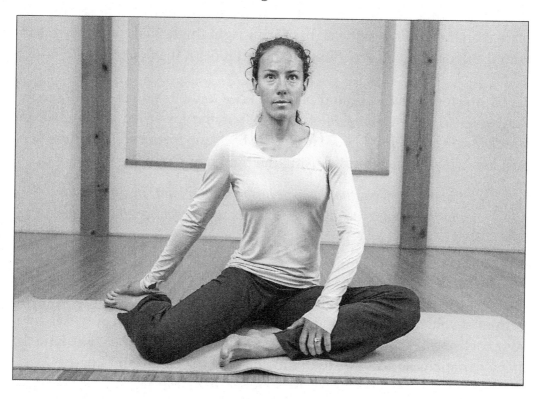

17. Lift the foot again and let the knee pass to the outside of the elbow and then continue lifting and lowering, each time passing the knee from inside to outside the elbow.

> *Make this movement smoother and more fluid each time by finding the movements in the hip joint, the trunk, and the scapula that allow the knee to pass the elbow.*

18. Let go of the right foot and rest.

19. Get a hold of the left foot and lift and lower it while passing the elbow to the inside and outside of the left knee.

20. The next time you lift the left foot, move it over to the right so you can place it on the ground to the right of your right thigh. Make a solid contact with the floor as if you are standing the left foot on the floor.

21. Lift the foot into the air and pass the knee to the inside of the left elbow until you can place the inside of the left foot and lower leg on the floor to your left side and behind you. Then move back and forth between these two positions slowly and carefully, using the right hand for support.

> *Feel the movements that happen inside the hip joint, in the trunk, and in the shoulder to allow the smoothest possible transition from place to place.*

22. Try the same movements on the right side. Each time you place the foot down on the ground, find a new place to rest it. You can place the foot more in front of you, to the left, to the right, or behind you. You can even roll onto your back and try to place the foot over your head or to either side. Find as many variations as possible, each time passing the elbow and knee.

Variations

Try holding the outsides of *both* feet with both hands, lifting the feet into the air, then passing the left knee to the inside of the left elbow, and placing the inside of the left foot behind you, at the same time you place the outside of the right foot in front of you. Then lift the feet into the air and reverse this so the right foot goes behind and the left foot comes in front. This will be difficult for most people so go very slowly!

You can also find many ways to hold the feet while rolling onto the back and then a to sitting position. Lesson 19 will give you some ideas.

17. Activating the Glutes

Purpose

To activate the glutes, a muscle group that many therapists and trainers believe is prone to inhibition. Most glute activation drills involve simply contracting them as hard as possible in one position, usually a bridge position. This lesson provides a wide variety of other positions and different types of contractions that will add value to any attempt to activate the glutes in functional activity. One or more of the movements below might be a useful part of a dynamic warmup for athletic activity.

Movements

1. Lie down on your back with your legs extended. Contract your glutes strongly on both sides several times. You can imagine you are trying to crack a nut between your glutes.

> *Note how the contraction of the glutes will raise your pelvis from the ground a little.*

> *How strong is the contraction? Use your hands to feel what parts of the glutes are contracting and which are not. Is it different from side to side?*

2. Contract just the right side and keep the left side fully relaxed. This will cause the right side of the pelvis to lift from the floor a little, so that your pelvis rolls to the left.

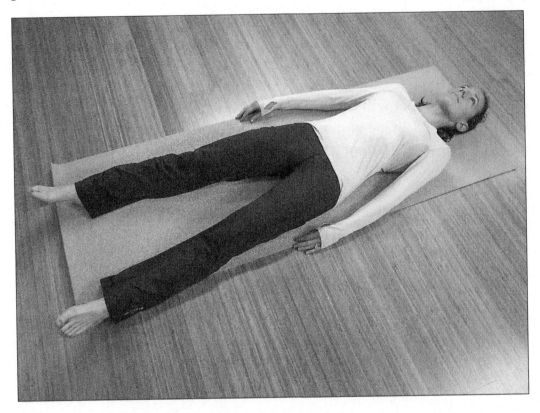

How long does it take for you to reach a full contraction of the pelvis?
How long does it take to fully relax it?

3. Contract and relax the right glute as quickly as possible, so your pelvis jumps on the right side and then falls.

4. Now contract and release the right-side glutes as *slowly* as possible so your pelvis rises and falls smoothly on the right side.

> *Do you find there are certain times when the movement speeds up quickly or becomes ratcheted and jerky? Try to smooth these out.*

5. Repeat these same movements on the left side while keeping the right side relaxed. Which side is easier to control? Which side has a stronger contraction?

6. Now move from side to side, contracting one set of glutes and then the other, so you roll from side to side. Try moving very slowly and smoothly and then very quickly and lightly.

7. Contract both glutes powerfully several times and note the strength and quality of the contraction. Do you notice any differences from the first time?

8. Here is a list of the different types of contractions we have tried so far:

* Maximum effort on both sides at the same time

* One at a time

* Back and forth

* Contract and relax as quickly as possible

* Contract and relax slowly and progressively

9. You can try each of these contractions in different positions. Each position will involve a different orientation of the hip joint which will emphasize different fibers of the glutes, stretch different tissues in the front of the hip (e.g. hip flexors and adductors), and have different effects on the knees, feet and spine. With that in mind, try the same movements in the following positions, while paying attention to the following finer points.

Kneeling

Come to a kneeling position so you are standing on your knees with your feet behind you. Focus on using the contraction of the glutes to bring the pubic bone up to the nose. (But not forward very much.) You can also think of lifting the navel.

> *Do you feel a strong stretch in the hip flexors? On which side do you feel a more intense stretch? When you contract the glutes on only one side, to which side does your pelvis turn? Can you do this with the abdominal muscles relaxed?*

Kneeling with knees wide and feet together

How is this position different from the previous one? Is the glute contraction stronger or weaker? This will probably change where you feel the stretch in the front of the hips. Note any differences from side to side.

Sitting with the soles of the feet together

In this position, it may be harder to feel the glutes contract. Repeat enough times to feel an improvement. Can you feel movement in the hip joint?

Half-kneeling

Stand on one knee with the opposite foot in front. Which glute is easier to contract? Which way does the pelvis want to turn? On which side do you feel more resistance from the hip flexors?

Standing

Stand with the feet about shoulder distance apart and turn the toes out slightly. Contract both glutes in standing a few times so you move the pubic bone up. How far does the pubic bone move forward? Can you contract the glutes and move the pubic bone up while not thrusting the pubic bone forward? What is the difference? What effect does this have on the curve in the low back? On the position of the chest?

Does the contraction of the glutes affect the position of the knees? Or the contact of the feet with the floor?

Make a strong connection to the ground with the ball of the big toe, the ball of the little toe, and the heel. Then contract the glutes and see if this causes the knees to turn out, and the inside arch of the foot to shorten and lift. Can you feel the connection between the activity of the glutes and the formation of the arch?

Squat

Assume the bottom position of the squat. Make a strong contact with the ball of the big toe, the ball of the little toe, and the heel and create an arch in the foot by rotating the knees outward and contracting the glutes. Once you can feel an isometric contraction of the glutes, use the glutes to move to a standing position by pushing the pubic bone forward and up. Finish in standing with a full contraction of the glutes and repeat.

After doing any of these variations, come to standing and take note of the level of tension in your low back. Walk around a little and feel the extension of the hip. Can you feel the glutes contracting to push the leg back? Can you feel hip flexors release to allow the leg to move back? Are there any differences between the right and left side?

18. Pelvic Clock

Purpose

To improve proximal control of the pelvis and to systematically identify and recover subtle movements of the pelvis that have been neglected.

Movements

1. Lie down on your back with your knees pointed to the ceiling and your feet on the ground. Arrange your feet so they are comfortably positioned and the hips joints are in a neutral position.

> *Feel the contact your pelvis makes with the floor. Where are the points of most pressure? Visualize the length of your spine from the tailbone, to the sacrum, to the curve of the low back, all the way to the neck.*

2. Imagine there is a clock painted underneath your pelvis. Twelve o'clock is somewhere near your low back, six o'clock is near your tailbone, three o'clock is approximately under the left hip joint, and nine o'clock is under the right hip joint.

3. Roll your pelvis on the floor away from you, so the point of heaviest pressure moves to six o'clock. You will feel your low back arching away from the floor. Then roll your pelvis back toward twelve o'clock so your low back presses into the floor. Repeat many times.

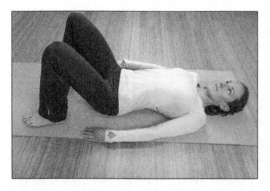 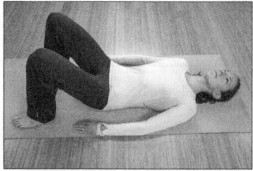

Make a smooth transition by keeping a slow, constant speed and a constant amount of pressure against the floor as you move.

4. Pause, and continue rolling, noting the contact of your head with the floor.

As you roll, does your head change its contact? Allow the neck and jaw to be free, so the head can respond to the movements of the pelvis.

As the pelvis rolls down to six o'clock, your head should roll down a little as well, so the chin comes closer to the chest. As the pelvis rolls back to twelve o'clock, it pushes the spine toward the head so it rolls up, and the chin tilts up toward the ceiling. Try to make sure any movements of the head are totally passive.

5. Pause.

6. Can you roll your pelvis from three o'clock to nine o'clock? In order to roll to three, the right side of the pelvis will lift a little from the floor, and you will roll your weight to the left. As you roll from three to nine, keep the line of pressure smooth and straight.

As you roll, do the knees tilt from side to side along with the pelvis? Try to keep the knees pointed to the ceiling. It is okay for the knees to move forward and back, but try to keep them pointed to the ceiling. This will require you to find some differentiated movement in the hip joints.

7. Continue to roll from three to nine. Do you roll the pelvis by pushing with the feet or pulling with the abdominal muscles? Try pressing into the floor with your right foot to roll the pelvis to the left and vice versa. Then, try rolling your pelvis from side to side while keeping a constant amount of pressure under the feet, so they cannot help. This would imply the movements of the pelvis are being controlled by the muscles above the pelvis in the stomach and low back. (You can try the same thing while rolling from twelve to six.)

8. Pause.

9. Can you roll around the clock in a clockwise direction? In other words, roll from one o'clock to two o'clock, etc. until you have made a circle.

> *Work very systematically and slowly to find the hours you tend to skip over, or places where you cannot apply pressure to the floor. Be very precise!*

> *You are trying to identify angles of movement you habitually avoid. Use your awareness and attention to restore control over movement at these angles.*

> *As you concentrate, make sure you're not holding your breath or creating excess muscular tension in your abs, hands, face or jaw.*

10. Pause.

11. Perform some circles counterclockwise and see if this affects your ability to hit each hour.

12. When you are becoming familiar with each minute of the clock, you can increase the speed of the circles, make them bigger or smaller, and try cutting through the clock at various diagonals.

13. As you circle the pelvis, can you feel other circles in your body? Does your head make a circle on the floor? Your navel? Your sternum? Can you feel alternating circular pressure under each scapula?

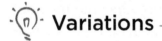 **Variations**

You can make similar clock movements in different positions.

On the back with soles of feet together

Lie on your back but instead of the feet standing on the floor, put the soles of the feet together so the knees hang out to the side. Performing clock movements in this position will place additional demands on mobility in the hip joint.

Sitting with soles of feet together

This can be done with the hands behind you for support, or leaning back onto the elbows for support. When you lean on your elbows, you'll find your clock is much bigger and there is more freedom of movement. Sitting with the hands for support requires greater control in the end range of hip flexion.

In either position, this is a good opportunity to pay attention to the integrated movements of the belly, sternum, and head as you move the pelvis. Notice that as the pelvis moves to six o'clock, the belly can expand forward, and you can inhale into the belly. Synchronize the breath so you exhale as the pelvis rolls back and allow the chest to collapse.

As you roll the pelvis to the left, notice that you may bring more weight into the right hand, and the head will tend to counterbalance by moving to the right.

As you circle the pelvis, note the circles that occur in the head, the navel, the sternum and the shoulder blades.

Sitting in a chair

Perform a few circles in your chair at work to bring some intelligence and awareness to the center of your body. Try to keep the head centered over the pelvis.

Standing

Imagine a light shining out of your pelvic floor and projecting directly onto the ground. (In case you don't have one already.) Draw circles on the floor. A good warm up for salsa dancing or belly dancing.

19. Rolling from the Back to Sitting

Purpose

To move through a fun developmental pattern that trains the function of the abductors and external rotators of the hip.

Movements

1. Sit with the soles of the feet together. Slide the right hand underneath the right heel so it can cup the heel. Take the left hand and grab the outside of the right foot from below. The thumb should be with the fingers.

2. Use the two hands to lift and lower the right foot. How heavy is the foot? How high does it go comfortably? Do you roll the pelvis back to make lifting easier?

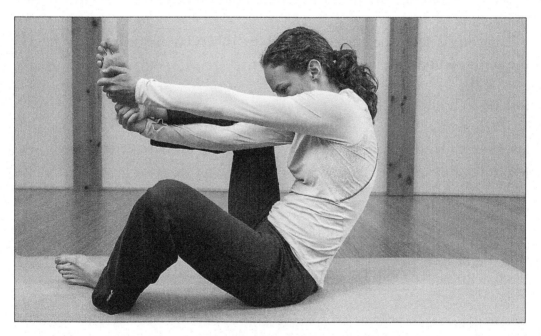

3. Pause and rest.

4. Bring the soles of the feet together again with both hands on the right foot as before.

5. Imagine there is a large pane of glass separating your two feet. Lift the right foot into the air and draw a large circle on the glass with the sole of the right foot. Move the foot toward you as you lift and away from you as you lower it.

Use the circle to loosen the hip. Allow the pelvis to roll and the spine to bend to allow the foot to move, so the circle becomes larger and larger. Change the direction of the circle and continue to expand its size.

6. Rest on your back with the soles of the feet together.

7. Get a hold of the right foot in the same way you did before, with the right hand holding the heel and the left hand holding the outside of the foot. Lift and lower the right foot high into the air. As the right foot lifts, lift the head at the same time, and then return it to the ground as the foot lowers.

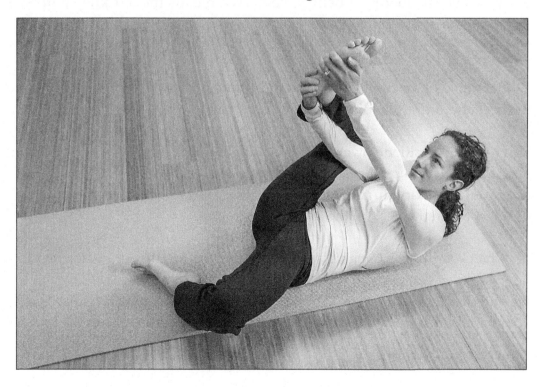

Feel how the front side of the body folds, and the low back presses more into the floor to support the lifting of the foot and head. How high can you lift the foot?

8. Pause.

9. Lift the foot a few more times, this time leaving the head on the floor. The next time you lift the right foot, move it over to the right so the right thigh and knee approach the floor. Then return. Repeat several times so you can feel the roundness of your back and develop a precise control of the speed of your rolling.

10. The next time the right upper leg touches the floor, can you find a way to roll into a side-sitting position? Try this a few times and see how it goes. Do you need a lot of momentum and oomph to get up? Let's work on that.

11. Come to sitting again with the right foot in the same position as before, but with the left foot bent behind you. That means the left knee will be somewhere near the right foot but the left lower leg will be pointing behind you, resting on its inside.

12. Get a hold of the right foot as you did before with the right hand cupping the heel and the left holding the outside of the foot.

13. From this position, lower your head down to the floor and then return. Each time you lower the head, let it hang down heavily until you reach your comfortable maximum range of motion. Feel the stretch in your right hip. Can you touch the head to the floor?

14. When your head is hanging as far to the floor as possible, or resting on the floor, sweep it from side to side, moving in an arc from the front of the right knee to the front of the right foot. Imagine you are sweeping the floor with your hair. Which part of the floor is easier to clean? Near the foot or the knee?

15. The next time your head sweeps to the right knee, continue to sweep the head along the ground *past* the knee and behind you until you find yourself rolling onto the right shoulder, and onto your back.

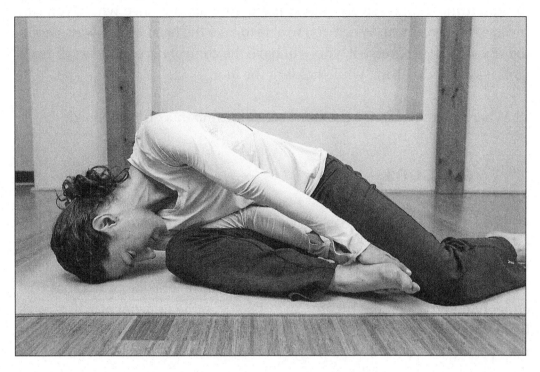

16. Now you should be on your back in the same position you were a moment ago, with the left knee hanging open, and holding the right foot with two hands. Can you reverse what you just did to come back to sitting?

17. You will bring the right foot over to the right until the knee hits the ground. *The key is to keep the head low over the right knee.*

> *Think about kissing the knee. This will load the muscles deep in the right hip. When they are fully loaded, they will activate to bring your spine to vertical with very little sense of voluntary effort. You can also use the right forearm and elbow to drive you up into the side-sitting position.*

18. If you are having trouble with this transition, simply return to the side-sitting position, lower the head to the ground, sweep it over to the right past the knee and then, *before you get to your back*, reverse the movement back to side sitting. Progressively extend the point past the knee where you can reverse the movement. When you're able to take the head all the way over to the right and still reverse it, you will have the control necessary to roll from your back to side sitting while holding the foot.

19. When you're ready, try the same set of movements on the left side.

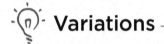 **Variations** ————————————————————————

You can roll from your back to side sitting in a similar manner with different grips on the foot. The hands could be reversed — the left hand holding the right heel and the right hand holding the outside of the foot.

You can also do this with only *one* hand on the outside of the foot. Try either hand on either foot. In any case, the key to the movement will always be to keep the head low over the elbow, knee and hip that provide the support to erect the spine up to sitting from lying down.

20. Rolling from the Stomach to Sitting

Purpose

A fun playful way to move from the stomach to sitting that integrates powerful hip extension and rotation with control of the trunk.

Movements

1. Lay down on your stomach. Place the palm of one hand on top of the other, and rest your right cheek on your hands so the head is turned to the left.

2. Bend the knees so the feet point to the ceiling and the lower legs are vertical. Join the knees and feet together as if they were tied with rope.

3. Keeping the knees and feet together, tilt the feet to the right in the direction of the floor. You will be pivoting on the right knee as the left knee comes off the floor.

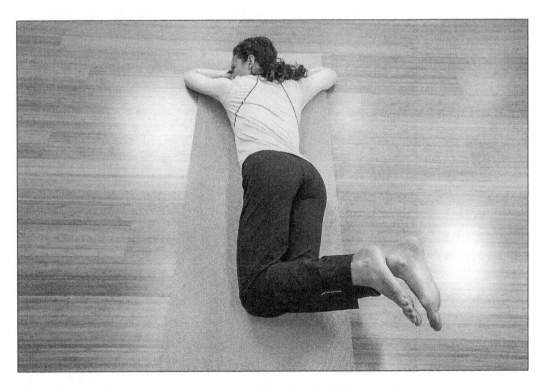

Find a comfortable range of motion for the feet to tilt. Feel the twist come into the ribs and spine. Repeat this many times to feel for what parts of your ribs, shoulder blades and spine need to soften to allow the knees to tilt easily.

4. Bring your feet back to the center. Turn your head to the right and tilt the knees over to the left a few times. Compare the ease of twisting on this side compared to the other one.

5. Bring your feet back to neutral and then tilt the knees to the right. Is it harder or easier than tilting them to the left? Go back and forth so you have a clear idea. Allow the shoulder blades to glide over the rib cage to allow the rib cage to turn and let the feet move.

6. Turn your head back to face the left. Tilt your legs over to the right a comfortable distance and let them stay there. Note their distance from the floor, if any.

7. Now, can you turn your head to the other side while keeping the legs in place? If not, allow the legs to move just a little to allow the head to turn. Then turn your head from side to side, leaving the legs in place.

8. Rest in any position that is comfortable.

9. Bring your hands to a pushup position. Turn your face to the left.

10. Tilt your knees over to the right and use your hands to help you turn and raise your head to look over your left shoulder to see the feet tilting toward the floor.

11. Synchronize the movement of the feet and head so that as soon as the feet begin to tilt, the head begins to lift and move in an arc to the left, until you can see over the left shoulder to the feet. Then lower the head and feet until they reach their starting position at the same time. The whole movement should feel integrated from head to foot.

12. Tilt the feet over to the right and lift the head to see them. When they are near the end range of motion, and when you can see them, start to slide the left knee away from the right knee along the right lower leg, until it rests on the floor just to the side of the right foot. As you do that, use the right hand to push yourself into a sitting position so you are sitting on the right buttock supported by the right hand.

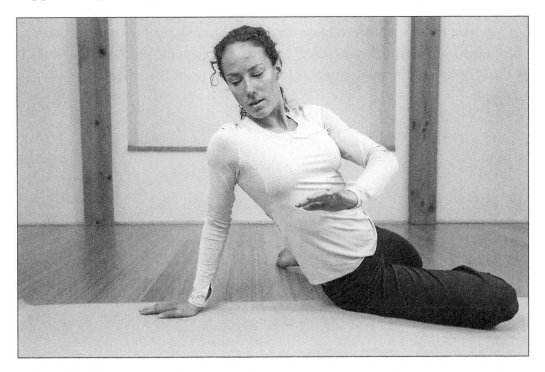

13. Now, can you smoothly return to your stomach by the same pathway? Look at the position of your right hand on the floor and imagine where the left hand needs to go to be in the same pushup position where you started. Then slowly slide the left hand into that position until you pull your chest to the floor and rotate the pelvis and the knees back to the starting position.

14. Then move back and forth between these two positions, each time making it more smooth and elegant and easy.

15. Try this on both sides. As you do, here are some tips to make the movement smoother. As the top leg slides away, use the glutes to "kick" the bottom

of the foot backward. The power of the leg helps pull you to sitting. Form a very solid contact with the hand that helps push you to sitting, and make sure it is in the most powerful position to help push.

16. As you return to the floor, keep the legs in position for as long as possible, until the chest pulls them passively back into position.

17. Once you become comfortable with the movement, play with transitioning from side to side as quickly as possible so you can use the momentum created by the legs to minimize any necessary pushing from the hands.

21. Crawling Part One

Purpose
To develop proximal control of the limbs in a locomotive pattern.

Movements
1. Come to your hands and knees. Try to arrange your hands so they are straight down from the shoulders and your knees so they are straight down from the hip joints. Lengthen your spine and balance your weight evenly on all four points of support.

2. Lift your right hand from the floor so your right shoulder moves closer to the ceiling. Imagine the arm is a limp rope, so all the muscles of the arm stay completely passive, and the movement is controlled from your trunk.

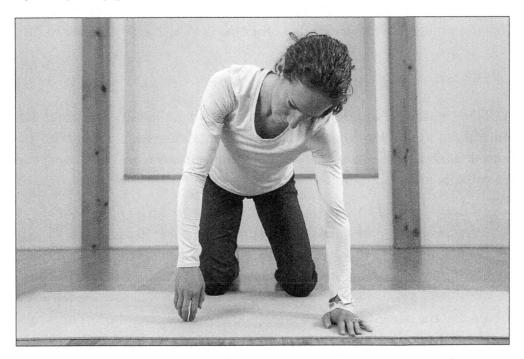

Allow your scapula to slide back and the chest to turn to the right as the right shoulder moves to the ceiling. Can you feel the weight shift to the left hand and knees as the right hand lifts?

3. Rest.

4. Repeat the same movement with the left arm a few times, again keeping it completely limp and passive like a rope. Allow your hand to slowly peel off the floor — the heel of the hand first and then the fingers. As the hand returns, the fingers touch first, then the heel.

5. Pause.

6. Now lift the right knee away from the floor by sending the back of the right hip to the ceiling. Keep the top of the right foot on the floor.

> *As with the arm, try not to use any muscles in the leg at all to create the movement. Feel how the pelvis rotates to lift the leg, and how your weight shifts to other points of support.*

7. Try the same movement with the other knee. Which side is easier to lift?

8. Pause.

9. Lift the right hand and right knee from the floor at the same time, and then return them to the floor many times. Make this movement as smooth and controlled as possible, so you are always moving at a slow constant speed, and you are not crashing into the ground as you return.

> *Notice you will have to shift your weight to the left to bring your center of mass over the points of support to the left. Try looking up and to the right as the right side lifts, and then down to the left hand as the left side comes back down to the ground.*

10. Now try the same movement on the other side, lifting the left hand and knee from the floor, while moving your support to the right hand and knee. Try to eliminate as much unnecessary muscle tension as possible as you do this. On which side do you have better balance?

11. Now alternate from side to side, lifting the right side, then the left. Once you have established a rhythm, step forward a few times, and then back. This is a homolateral pattern of crawling, where one hand works with the same side knee.

12. Pause.

13. Lift the right hand away from the floor at the same time as the left knee, so each limb dangles like a rope. Hold them both in place at their highest point so you can feel the muscle activity in the trunk that creates the counter rotation between the shoulders and hips.

14. Do the same thing on the opposite hand and foot and compare. Which diagonal feels more natural?

15. The next time you lift both the right hand and the left knee, step forward with each, and then the opposite diagonal, so you are crawling forward in a contralateral pattern.

> *Keep a minimum of muscular activity in the arms and legs, so the movement is mostly controlled from the center of your body. Imagine the slow powerful movements of a lion stalking prey.*

16. Crawl forward and back, fast and slow. Keep your head free to look at the horizon and turn from side to side. Can you find a way to move immediately into a side-sitting position in the middle of your crawling? (Hint: Watch a baby; they do this constantly.)

17. When you are ready, stand up and walk around a little. Notice the cross-lateral pattern used in walking — how the right shoulder moves back at the same time the left hip moves back. Can you feel how the center of the body can control the movements of the arms and legs, so they respond like passive ropes to the powerful large muscles in the center of the body?

22. Crawling Part Two

Purpose

To use some unique movements in the crawling position to challenge the performance of the deep hip muscles in providing stability and balance.

Movements

1. Come to your hands and knees.

2. Slide the right knee forward and then to the left, so you can sweep the right foot around the left knee and then down, until the right knee comes to rest just to the outside the left knee.

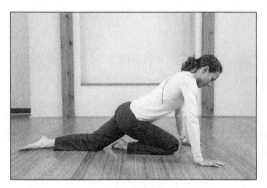 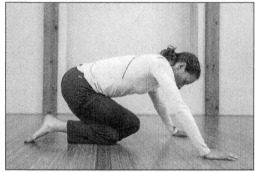

3. Then slide back to the starting position and move back and forth many times.

4. As you slide, make sure the right knee, lower leg and top of the foot stay on the floor so you are not lifting them.

> *Notice that your left hip must provide balance and support for the right knee to be free to move. Can you feel the muscles in the back of the left hip working?*

5. Now try the same movement with the opposite knee. Slide the left knee forward until the left foot moves into the gap between the right hand and the right knee, and then slide the left knee until it is snug against the outside of the right knee.

As the knee comes forward, does your head look down or up? Try it both ways. Each time the knee slides forward, look up, and each time it slides back look down.

Then try the reverse. Which is more natural?

6. Come to neutral and rest.

7. Slide the right knee back on the floor and to the left until it can pass *behind* the left foot, and then come back up until it is snug to the outside of the left knee. Then slide back to the starting position and repeat this movement many times.

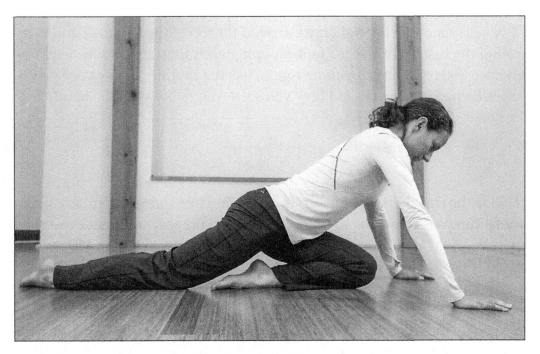

As before, always keep the knee and lower leg and foot on the ground as it slides, so you are not lifting. Feel the pelvis rock back to help you clear the foot. Feel the stretch and the work of the muscles in the back of the left hip.

8. Rest.

9. Try the same movement on the other side so you slide the left knee down below the right foot and up to the outside of the right knee.

10. After a few repetitions, add in the first movement by sliding the left knee around the right knee to the front. So you slide the left knee in a full circle all the way around the right foot and the right knee.

> *As you do the movement, notice whether your head goes up or down as the knee slides. Is there a pattern? Coordinate the entire spine in the movement.*

11. Pause.

12. Now try moving the right knee around the top of the left knee, and then around the bottom of the left foot, stopping each time at the outside of the left knee and reversing direction. Again, feel the rhythm of how your pelvis moves forward and back, and how you shift weight between the hands and the knee.

13. Pause.

14. Slide the right knee up and around the left. Then slide the left knee *down* until it can pass below the right foot to come all the way up to slide over the top of the right knee and rest to its outside. Then repeat the same movement on the other side so you are advancing forward. Move the hands as necessary to crawl forward in this rather bizarre manner.

15. Try to find the best time to advance the hand forward so it always provides a perfect counterbalance to the movement of the knees. Just as in normal crawling, it will probably be easiest to move one hand forward at the same time the opposite knee is moving forward.

16. Can you crawl backward this way as well?

23. Coordinating the Foot and Ankle

Purpose

To coordinate complex rotational and tilting movements of the subtalar joint with movements at the ankle, knee and hip. **Note: You might feel some foot cramps in this lesson. Pause until the cramping is over, then continue.**

Movements

1. Lie on your stomach and place your forehead on your hands. Bend your knees so the lower legs point to the ceiling.

2. Make sure the lower legs are truly vertical, not tilted to one side or the other.

3. Arrange the soles of your feet so they are parallel to the ceiling, as if they're standing on the ceiling. You can take a look back to see how well you did.

4. Join the knees, ankles and feet together, so the knees are touching, the inside of the heels are touching, and the balls of the big toes are touching.

5. Flex and extend the ankles many times while keeping the balls of the big toes and heels touching. Do you feel cramping in the foot muscles?

6. Keep the big toes and knees together but move the heels away from each other. Bring them back and repeat this movement many times.

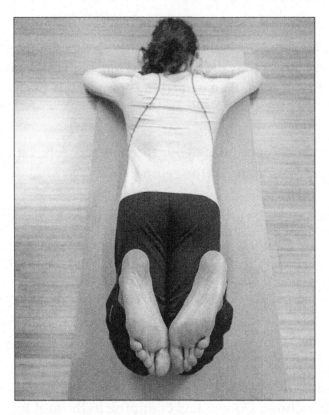

Can you do this movement smoothly and easily or does it feel labored and effortful? What muscles can you feel working to create this movement?

7. Now reverse the movement so the heels stay together, but the toes move away from each other. Which movement is easier? Alternate between the two movements to find out. See if you can transition from one movement to the other smoothly.

8. Try the same alternating movement with the right foot only, keeping the left foot still. Switch sides so only the left foot moves. Which side is easier to coordinate?

9. Sit in a chair with your feet flat on the floor. Sense how your right foot makes contact with the floor. Notice in particular the quality of contact with the heel, the ball of the big toe, and the ball of the little toe.

10. Imagine the ball of the right big toe is pinned to the ground. Keep it pinned and rotate your right heel to the right and left by sliding the heel on the floor.

> *Which direction is easier? Can you feel this movement in your knee? In your hip?*

11. Now pin the heel to the floor and slide the toes inward and outward.

> *How does the contact of your foot change as you rotate the foot? What is the effect on the arch?*

12. Bring the right foot back to neutral. Then tilt your right knee to the inside and outside, so you roll onto the inside and outside of the right foot.

13. Now try to tilt the knee back and forth *while keeping the right foot flat on the floor*. Make sure the balls of the big and little toes stay in firm contact with the floor as the knee tilts.

14. How about the reverse? Can you tilt the right foot from the inside to the outside edge while keeping the knee fixed in the exact same place?

15. Return to the movement of pinning the heel and rotating the toes. Can you feel the foot tilt from side to side as you rotate? As you rotate the toes inward, which side of the foot comes away from the floor? Can you keep that side down even as you rotate inward? Keep the balls of the big and little toes in solid contact with the floor as you slide them left and right.

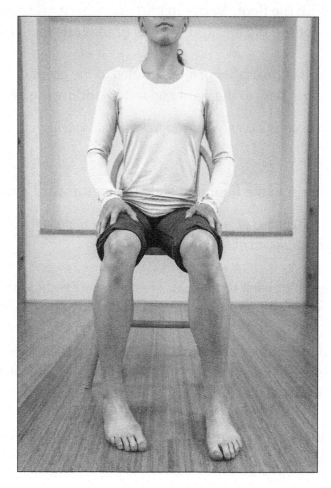

Can you feel the muscles in the arch of your foot working as you do this?

16. Stand facing a few feet from a wall with your hands resting lightly on the wall.

17. Pin the ball of your right big toe to the ground and rotate your heel to the inside and outside. Try to keep your pelvis pointed directly at the wall so it does not rotate with the foot.

> *Sense the movement that occurs in the hip joint. Where do you feel the movement occurring? Is it easier to rotate in or out?*

18. Now pin the heel and rotate the toes in and out. Is this easier or harder than rotating the heel?

19. Can you keep your foot in neutral (no tilting one side up and down) as you rotate in and out?

20. Walk around or perform other movements like squatting to compare the quality of movement at the right ankle, knee and hip to the left. Can you sense any differences? Repeat this lesson on the left side to even things out.

24. Improving the Squat

Purpose

To improve the squat! But in an indirect way. Children learn to squat as a transitional position between sitting and standing.

All the movements in this lesson are based around a position where you have your hands and feet flat on the floor. I will refer to this as the "four point" position. It is also sometimes called a bear crawling position.

Each part of the lesson involves performing some movement in this position or transitioning in or out of this position. Once you are familiar with each part, put them together in creative ways. Together, the movements make an excellent part of a warmup for exercise.

Note: Unlike the other lessons, this one may cause some fatigue. Fatigue is okay, as long as there is no pain and fatigue does not compromise your ability to control movement or pay attention to your movement. This lesson is also far longer than the others. So until it is familiar, it is best to practice only one or two parts at a time.

Assessment

Before starting the lesson, assess your current level of function by squatting down as far as you can go while keeping your heels on the floor. How far down did you go? Can you rest your pelvis on your heels? How long could you stay in this position comfortably? How much can you do in this position? Can you turn your head to see behind you, reach things on the ground, or shift your weight from foot to foot?

Although this lesson does not directly train the squat, you may find that your function in this position changes after practicing the lesson.

Movements

1. To start the lesson, come to a standing position. Make sure your shoes are off. Spread your feet a comfortable distance apart.

2. Lower your hands to the ground until you can place them flat on the ground in front of you. Then rise to a standing position and then move back and forth between these two positions many times.

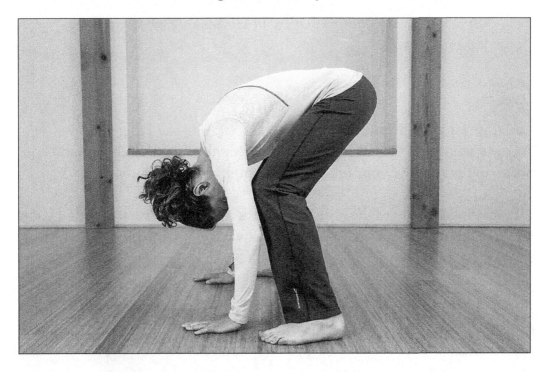

3. You can bend at the knees as much as you want, but keep the heels flat on the ground. If you can't, then find a way to "raise the ground" by using an elevated surface for the hands.

4. With your hands flat on the ground, you have four points of support. Note the relative positions of the four points. Throughout the lesson, continue to adjust and refine the positions of the four points to make your movements more comfortable and easy.

You can try the feet farther apart, closer together, turned in or turned out. Same thing with the hands. You can also play with the weight distribution between the hands and feet. Find the right angle to bend the knees. Is it better to let the head hang down or hold it up?

5. Repeat the movement, constantly changing all these variables until the most efficient way to optimize all the movement starts to emerge.

> *How would you do this movement if you had to do it all day long? (By the way, you did this movement all day long when you were learning to walk.)*

6. Rest.

Looking around in four points

1. Lower your hands to the ground again. Keep the hands on the ground and notice the position of your four points of support. Get comfortable.

2. From here, look up to the horizon, and then down and back between your legs so you can look behind you. Move back and forth between these two positions many times.

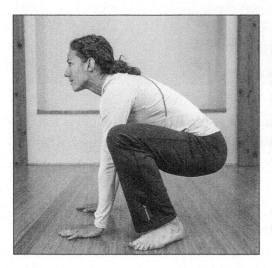 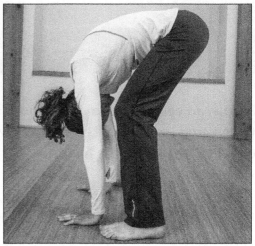

3. Rest in standing or sitting, whichever you prefer.

> *As you look between your legs, raise your pelvis as high as you can and feel a stretch in the hamstrings. As you look up, lower your pelvis as far as possible to challenge the mobility in your hips, chest and ankles.*

4. Return to four points and repeat the same movements, looking up to the horizon and down between your legs.

> *Notice that there is an inverse relationship between the head and pelvis — as one rises, the other falls.*

> *Continue to refine the placement of your feet and hands to increase your range of motion. Don't push through your resistance, just explore where the resistance is, and wait for it to move.*

5. Rest in standing or sitting.

6. Come to four points again, and note the weight distribution on your feet. Does your weight fall to the inside or outside? Equalize the weight distribution and form a strong contact in the shape of the tripod — the ball of the big toe, the ball of the little toe and heel. Make a similar contact with the hands.

7. Start looking to the right and to the left and behind you if possible.

> *Notice how your pelvis and spine needs to participate in the movement to give you a good view. Feel the movement in the ribs, ankles and feet. The whole body cooperates.*

8. Rest for a moment and return to the movement, scanning to the right and left on the horizon and the ground.

> *Notice how the pressure under the feet changes as you turn. Do you feel like one heel wants to leave the floor?*

9. Rest.

Reaching in four points

1. Come to the four points position.

2. Imagine you want to paint the floor with the palm of your right hand, and you want to cover as much ground as possible, but your feet and other hand

are nailed to the floor. Try to paint the space in front of you, to either side, between your legs, and behind you.

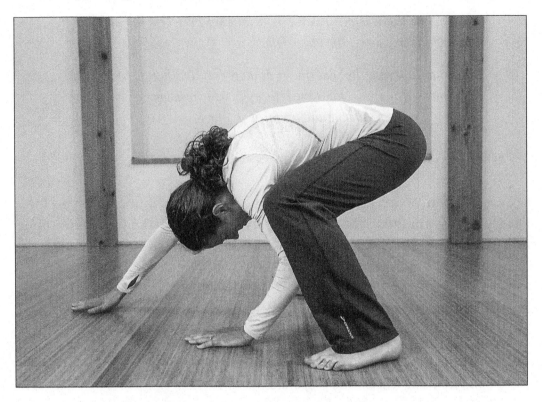

3. Feel how the powerful muscles of the hips and thighs support and balance your weight. Can you feel how even small movements of the pelvis cause a large stretch?

4. Rest.

> *Note your level of fatigue and stay within your limits. Learn how to make the work easier not harder. You did similar movements all day as a toddler. You weren't fitter then, just more efficient.*

5. When you are ready, return to the four points position again and start painting the floor with the left hand. Reach to all sides of your body.

Notice that this is a movement of your whole body, involving coordinated activities in the feet, ankles, knees, hips, spine, ribs, and shoulders.

6. Rest.

7. Return to four points and then paint the floor with both hands at the same time. You can move the hands together, apart, or in large circular patterns. Try making solid contact with the whole palm of the hand so you press a little into the floor. Keep your shoulders well away from your ears and the neck long and free.

8. Rest.

Shifting weight and walking

1. Come to four points.

2. Lift just the right hand from the floor and put it back down.

Lift the hand as if the arm was a rope, so the heel of the hand comes off first, and then the fingers last. Lift the fingers until they barely leave the floor, just a paper's width, then return all your weight to the right hand, so you are pawing the floor very softly.

3. Rest in sitting.

4. Return to four points and begin lifting and lowering the left hand in the same manner, keeping the arm like a rope.

What do you do to lift the hand? Play with different ways to lift the hand and find out how to make the movement of the hand as light and sensitive as possible. The more parts of yourself you can involve, particularly the pelvis, the better the quality of the movement.

5. Now alternate lifting the right hand and then the left, so you are pawing back and forth. Find a rhythm.

You might feel your pelvis rocking from side to side, the weight shifting from foot to foot. Feel how many powerful muscles in our body are engaged by this simple movement.

6. Rest.

7. Return to four points.

8. Now lift the right foot from the floor and place it back down again and do this many times.

How smooth and quiet can you make the lifting and lowering of the right foot? Imagine you had a scale under the right foot and you wanted the numbers to rise and fall smoothly as opposed to gyrating wildly up and down.

9. Rest in sitting.

10. Return to four points.

11. Lift the left foot several times.

Where does your weight shift? To the right hand? The left hand? The left foot?

12. Now alternate — lift the right foot then the left, trying to keep the hands on the ground as much as possible. Let the feet rise and fall as softly as possible.

13. Rest, then come to the four points position again.

14. Lift the right foot and right hand at the same time and then place them back to the ground gently.

Feel how you need to shift weight onto the left side, especially the left hip. Notice if you are able to lower the right foot and hand with control or if they crash to the ground.

15. Now lift the left hand and left foot and set them down. Try to raise and lower the hand and foot at exactly the same time.

16. Alternate from side to side, so you lift the right foot and hand, then the left foot and hand, so you are rocking back and forth from side to side.

17. Rest.

18. Return again and start marching back and forth. Keep the rhythm and use this pattern to start walking forward. So the right hand and foot move forward together and then the left foot and left hand move forward. And walk back to where you started and march in place a little.

19. Now use the same pattern to walk a little left like a crab by widening and shortening your stance. Then walk back to where you started.

20. Rest.

21. Come to the four points position again.

22. Now lift the right foot and the left hand at the same time. So you are lifting on a diagonal. This might be difficult. Take your time and you will get it.

> This might be easier if you imagine it differently — instead of thinking of lifting the right foot and left hand, imagine pressing in and supporting yourself with the left foot and right hand.

23. Rest.

24. Now try the opposite pair — lift the left foot and the right hand from the ground at the same time. If you cannot fully lift the foot or hand, just make it lighter on the floor.

25. Now alternate — lift the left foot and right hand, then the right foot and left hand. Feel the rhythm, the movements that need to happen in the shoulders as the weight shifts.

26. Now keep this pattern and use it to walk forward. Then walk back.

27. Rest.

28. Come to four points position again.

29. Lift both hands so you rock back to the feet. Now lift both feet by rocking to the hands.

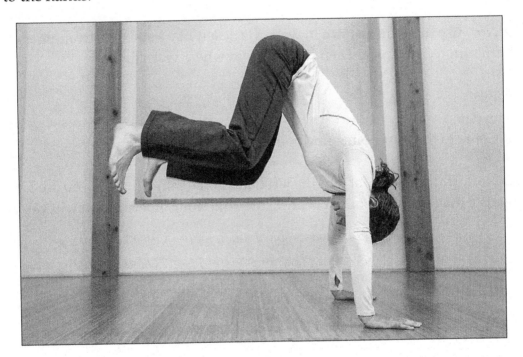

30. Now lift all four at the same time. You can do it. (Hint: jumping.) Jump a few times but stay within your limits.

31. Now use any pattern you want — homolateral, cross-lateral, crab or jumping to move around right, left, or sideways like a monkey.

32. Rest.

33. Walk around a little and feel the connection between your arms and legs with your trunk as you walk, how they all pull through the center of the body. See if you can recall any of the sensations of moving on the ground as a four-legged animal.

Transition to side sitting

1. Come to four points again.

2. Look at the space between your right hand and right foot and draw a line between them. Then lift the left foot, allow the left knee to bend, and place the left knee on the ground somewhere in the middle of the line between the right foot and hand. Keep the right foot and both hands on the ground.

3. If you have put the left knee in the correct place then you will be resting on the left buttock and the outside of the left thigh and you will be looking to the horizon over to the right. Notice that the right foot is still planted on the ground as are both hands. The left foot will end up somewhere near the right foot.

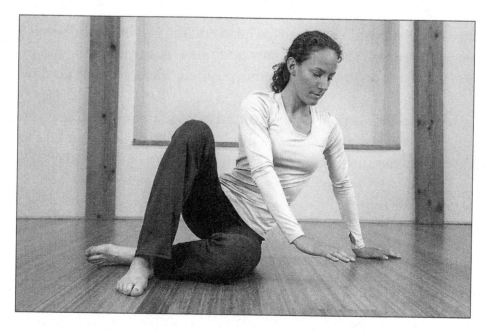

4. Now from this position, return to the four points again by lifting the left knee from the ground and placing it back to its original position. Now go back and forth between these positions several times so that you are alternating between four points, and sitting with the left knee to the right.

5. Notice what happens with the right foot, the supporting foot. Does it pivot or rotate outward to the right as you spiral down? Does the heel rise to make the pivot easier? You can experiment with leaving it in place and see if you can sit that way, but it's fine to let it move as well.

6. Rest. If you had any trouble with that movement, you can try a very similar movement from your hands and knees, which is much easier.

7. Now lets do the same on the other side. Bring the right knee to rest on the floor between the left foot and left hand, then return to four points and go back and forth.

8. Notice the trajectory of the pelvis as you move. As you sit, the pelvis comes down and turns left. As you move to four points, the pelvis rises and turns to face front. It's a spiral.

9. Notice the relationship between the head and the pelvis. As the pelvis goes down to the ground, the head comes up to look at the horizon, and as the pelvis comes back up to the four points position, the head must go down.

10. Try to make your arrival on the ground as smooth as possible so you are touching down very lightly. You can think of lightly kissing your butt to the ground and then returning.

11. Rest.

12. Come to four points again.

13. Try to alternate the same movement from side to side. You sit to the left, then come back to four points and then sit to the right.

14. Find a rhythm so you have very smooth transitions. As you move, notice which hand becomes lighter on the ground. For example, as you face the right, which hand becomes light enough on the ground that you could actually lift from the ground?

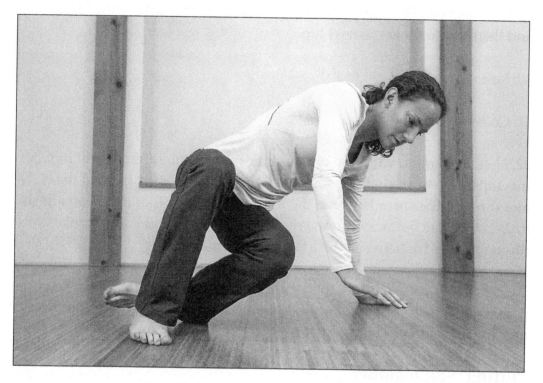

15. Start to lift one hand from the ground as you go down and return that hand to the ground as you come to the middle point, then lift the other hand as you go to the other side.

16. Rest.

17. Return to four points and move from side to side again. Start to move faster, so your butt is lightly kissing down on the ground as you move from side to side.

18. As you transition through the four points position, you can actually hop from foot to foot to give the movement more bounce and speed. So as you

rise from the left side on the power of the left foot, you can then jump your weight over to the right foot, and then go down on the right side, so you are hopping from side to side.

19. Feel how you are really loading up each hip like a spring and releasing and then loading into the next hip.

20. Rest.

21. Come to four points.

22. Here is a similar variation on the same movement. Lift the right foot but this time keep the right knee somewhat extended, so you can send the right foot through the space between the left hand and left foot until you are sitting on the right buttock with the right leg fully extended out in front of you through the space between the left hand and foot.

23. Practice this a few times, then try transitioning left to the right. You can jump from side to side as you did before. This may have the feel of break dancing or caoeria.

Putting it all together

How many different ways can you find to combine all these movements? Play around with all these for five to twenty minutes as an excellent warm up for exercise or a great standalone workout.

25a. Sitting in a Chair Part One

Purpose

To sit with more comfort and ease.

Note: It will helpful (but not necessary) to sit on a chair that is hard and flat.

Movements

1. Sit at the front of your chair with your feet flat on the floor, hands on your knees. Sense your overall level of comfort, ability to breathe, and your ability to turn to look right or left.

2. Feel the contact of your sit bones with the chair. (The sit bones are the bony projections at the bottom of your pelvis. You can use your hands to feel them.)

3. Roll your pelvis forward and back on the sit bones so you can sense their shape. Notice the parts that are round, pointy, narrow, thick, angled upward or downward. Sense the amount of weight on the left compared to the right. Equalize the weight.

4. Expand your range of motion, finding how far you can roll forward and back.

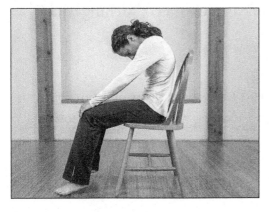 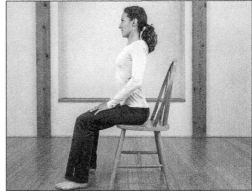

5. Continue to roll the pelvis forward and back and place one hand on the low back. Notice that as the pelvis rolls forward, the low back arches and the vertebrae come forward. As you roll backward, the low back rounds and the vertebrae push backward. Feel the change as you roll forward and back. Feel the low back muscles tightening and relaxing as you roll.

6. Continue to roll and place your fingers on your navel. As the pelvis rolls forward, allow the belly to expand and the navel to move forward. As the pelvis rolls backward, allow the belly to contract and the navel to move backward. Inhale into the belly as it expands and exhale as the belly contracts.

7. Continue to roll and place your fingers on the middle of your sternum. As the pelvis rolls forward, allow the chest to expand and the sternum to move forward and up. As the pelvis rolls back, allow the chest to slump and the sternum to move down and back. Breathe into the chest as it expands; exhale as it slumps.

8. Continue to roll. As the pelvis rolls back, move your head and eyes to look at your navel. As you roll the pelvis forward, move your head and eyes to look at the ceiling above you.

9. Continue to roll and notice your whole spine is arching and rounding. Which parts round the most? Which arch the most? Try to make the curves smooth and symmetrical so each part of the spine is rounding or arching equally.

10. Pause.

11. Place a hand on the crown of your head to monitor your height. Continue to roll while keeping your head level and looking toward the horizon.

12. Notice that your height changes as you roll forward and back. As you roll back, your pelvis will lose height and you will get shorter. As you roll forward, you will lengthen for a while until you roll off the sit bones onto the hamstrings and then you will start to get shorter again. (Note: getting shorter requires a larger range of motion and is harder to notice.)

13. Reduce your range of motion until you are moving a smaller and smaller distance around either side of the tallest point on your sit bones. Stop at the tallest point and remove your hand from your head.

14. Assess your overall level of comfort, ability to breathe, and ability to turn to look left or right. Feel the length of the spine and the height through the crown of the head. Are you sitting taller with more ease?

25b. Sitting in a Chair Part Two

Purpose

To sit with more comfort and adaptability.

Movements

1. Sit to the front of your chair with your feet flat on the floor, hands on your knees. Assess your overall level of comfort, ability to breathe, and your ability to turn to look left or right.

2. Sense your contact with the chair. Which sit bone bears more weight?

3. Lift the left sit bone from the chair by shifting weight onto the right sit bone. Repeat several times. Does your head and body lean over to the right like a tower? Try to keep your head centered over your pelvis. This means your left side will have to shorten.

4. To feel the left side shorten, put your left hand on your waist with the thumb to the back and the fingers to the front. Feel your left hip hiking to the ribs, the left waist shortening, and the muscles under your hand contracting.

5. Move to the left of your seat until the left sit bone is hanging over the chair and you are supported only by the right sit bone. Let the left sit bone drop toward the floor below the level of the chair and then raise it above the level of the chair. Repeat several times. Feel the left side alternatingly lengthen and shorten.

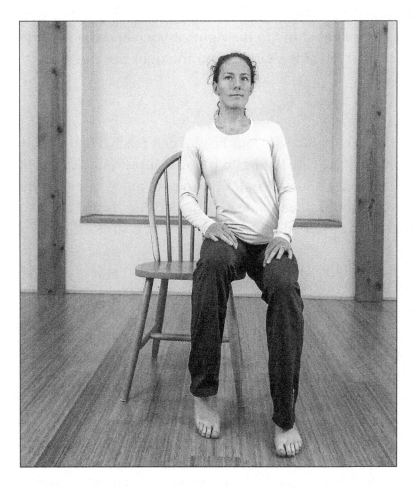

6. Move back to the middle of your seat. Put your left hand on the crown of your head and pull your left elbow in the direction of the left hip. How does your weight shift on the sit bones? To the left or the right? Move in such a way that the weight shifts to the right sit bone and the left lifts from the chair.

7. Notice each time the head comes down, the right ribs expand and the left ribs contract like an accordion.

8. Reach your arms out directly to the sides so they are like a scarecrow. Reach the right arm farther to the right while keeping the arms level. How does your weight shift on the sit bones? To the left or the right? Do they move in such a way that the weight shifts to the right sit bone and the left lifts from the chair. Notice your left side shortens and the right ribs push out to the right.

9. Pause.

10. Extend the right hand over your head. Then reach it to the ceiling as high as possible as if you were trying to pick an apple. How does your weight shift on the sit bones? Guess what? Once again, move in such a way that the weight shifts to the right sit bone and the left lifts from the chair. Feel the ribs on the right expand and the ribs on the left contract.

11. Repeat some of the same movements on the left side.

12. Reach your right arm to the ceiling and then the left arm, one after the other. Notice your weight shifts from one sit bone to the other. Use this movement to let your sit bones march in place from side to side.

13. With your hands at your sides, march the sit bones in place, lifting one or the other. Lift each one less and less until the weight is equal on both.

14. Place your hands on your knees again. March your sit bones in place, and then try to walk them a few steps to the front of the chair and then a few steps to the back. Try to keep your head and shoulders relatively quiet, so they stay balanced over the pelvis and most of the movement happens below the chest.

15. When you are done, reassess your comfort in your chair. Does your pelvis feel more alive?

Repetition and Progression: Moving On

Now that you have tried some or all of the lessons, what next?

The answer will be different depending on your goals and your status. But here are some general ideas for repeating and progressing the lessons, and making sure the benefits transfer into your activities of everyday life or sports.

* The lessons can be progressed by following the variations, making up your own, and performing the movements more quickly. Aside from the squat, most of the specific movements used in the lessons are not well-suited to loading with resistance or repeating in a way that will create exercise stress. However, each of the movements, if improved in some way, will likely transfer to other movements that are used in exercise. For example, although I would not recommend you start crawling long distances to get fit, the cross-lateral patterns of movement that can be improved by crawling might improve your running gait, and make you more capable of loading this movement.

* For any lesson, or particular movement in a lesson, repeat it as often as you have the interest, focus and ability to improve it in some way. If a movement or lesson does not seem to offer any perceptible benefit, don't repeat it over and over. Try something else. Maybe come back to it later.

* In trying to determine how often to repeat lessons that are helpful, consider the four different types of neuroplastic changes discussed earlier in the book.

* Maintaining good habits of movement that are already well developed may take just a few minutes of "activation" work every other day. This might involve nothing more than performing some squatting, rolling, reaching, rotating or crawling movements. These movements might

make an excellent part of a movement prep or warmup to vigorous exercise, or as a quick refreshing break from sitting during the day. For many people, an active lifestyle or exercise program that involves fundamental movements will be sufficient to maintain healthy patterns of movement all by itself.

* Trying to recover basic patterns of movement that have been neglected for a while will take more time and effort. Building new patterns of movement will take even longer.

* The most difficult task is to break maladaptive *habits* of movement, such as creating excess tension or perceiving excess threat. Chronic pain often involves these habits. Persistence, optimism, resourcefulness, and guidance from a qualified expert may be necessary to break them. Remember that not all pain has a movement solution.

* If you find the benefits of a lesson are temporary, and therefore require repeating, this would imply that the neural patterns of movement or perception that are invoked by the lesson are "fragile." They are not yet permanent, or they are in competition with some other movement pattern that is more habitual.

* To make the benefits of any lesson more permanent, repeat it enough times so you are familiar with the basic movements, then experiment with trying to get the same benefit in far less time. For example, in the rolling lessons, you may find that after some practice, you can obtain their full benefit in just thirty seconds of rolling from side to side.

* Another way to integrate the benefits of any lesson into everyday life is to be very aware of how your body is moving differently after the lesson, in as many contexts as possible. For example, if your shoulder feels better aligned and more comfortable after a particular lesson, how does this affect the way it feels when you are walking? When you are lifting weights? When you are reaching for a computer mouse? Is

there an activity that prompts you to revert to your older, more stressful habits of using the shoulder?

* Often, exposure to excess stress in the form of vigorous exercise, prolonged postures, or negative emotions will prompt us to abandon newer patterns of movement and revert to old habits. The earlier you can recognize a bad habit reemerging, the better able you will be to inhibit it and maintain a newer, more desirable habit. In other words, increased mindfulness and awareness of your movement throughout the day is the best way to integrate any beneficial changes from these lessons.

* If you feel like you are walking taller or with better posture after a particular lesson, does this remain true even after you run many miles? If your shoulder feels free from habitual tension after the shoulder clock lesson, does it stiffen after some heavy bench presses? If you find yourself reverting back to habitual, protective ways of moving after the stress of exercise or anything else, it is useful to be aware of this breaking point and what causes it. Progress involves extending that point out farther through a process of graded exposure and progressive overload, which are the cornerstones any successful program of exercise.

Best of luck!

RESOURCES

FOR FURTHER INFORMATION related to this book, including articles and audio movement lessons, visit bettermovement.org and guidetobetter movement.com.

ABOUT THE AUTHOR

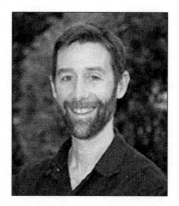

TODD HARGROVE lives in Seattle with his wife and two daughters.

He is a Certified Rolfer and Feldenkrais Practitioner and helps clients move better and feel better in private sessions and classes.

For more information visit his blog at bettermovement.org or the website for this book at guidetobettermovement.org.

ENDNOTES

[1]   Weepier, Magnusson (2010) Increasing Muscle Extensibility: A Matter of Increasing Length or Modifying Sensation? *Physical Therapy,* March 2010, Vol. 90, No. 3, 438–449; http://www.physther.net/content/90/3/438.full

[2]   Chaudry, Schleip (2008) Three-Dimensional Mathematical Model for Deformation of Human Fasciae in Manual Therapy. *J Am Osteopath Assoc.* August 1, 2008, Vol. 108, No. 8, 379–390; http://www.jaoa.org/content/108/8/379.full

[3]   This book does not discuss the precise ranges of motion, sequences of joint movement, or muscle activation patterns that should be present in a forward bend, overhead reach, or squat. While this specific and focused approach to analyzing movement is very useful, it has some weaknesses. First, it relies on measurements that can be inaccurate or hard to make. Many movement assessments simply do not measure what we think they do. Second, it is based on anatomical research that is unclear and subject to change. For example, world class anatomists are still debating if the trapezius upwardly rotates the scapula and if the psoas contributes to anterior pelvic tilt. Third, these approaches may not take into account anatomical or structural differences between individuals. What is right for one person might be wrong for another.

[4]   Tyler, et al. (2001) The Association of Hip Strength and Flexibility With the Incidence of Adductor Muscle Strains in Professional Ice Hockey Players. *American Journal of Sports Medicine,* Vol. 29, No. 2.

[5]   Trehearn, Burghs, et al. (2009) Sit-and-reach flexibility and running economy of men and women collegiate distance runners. *J Strength Cond Res.* 2009 Jan. 23; http://www.ncbi.nlm.nih.gov/pubmed/19050648

6   Mok, Brauer, Hodges (2007) Failure to use movement in postural strategies leads to increased spinal displacement in low back pain. *Spine* (Phila Pa, 1976). 2007 Sep 1; 32(19); http://www.ncbi.nlm.nih.gov/pubmed/17762795

7   Cook (2010) Movement; Sahrmann (2002) Diagnosis and Treatment of Movement Impairment Syndromes; McGill (2007) Low Back Disorders; Page, Frank (2010) *Assessment and Treatment of Muscle Imbalance: The Janda Approach.*

8   Feldenkrais (2009) *Awareness Through Movement.*

9   Francis, Charlie, High Octane Training: Q&A for high-performance athletes. Article in *T-Nation.* http://www.tnation.com/free_online_article/ sports_body_training_performance/high_octane_training;jsessionid= 27A6043C50F641D85CF03EDC35877306-mcd02.hydra

10   Shumway-Cook, Woolacott (2012) *Motor Control: Translating Research into Clinical Practice,* 4th Ed. p. 31.

11   Shumway-Cook, Woolacott (2012) p. 31.

12   Shumway-Cook, Woolacott (2012) p. 13–16; Bernstein (1996) *On Dexterity and Its Development.*

13   Christensen, Hartvigsen (2008) Spinal curves and health: a systematic critical review of the epidemiological literature dealing with associations between sagittal spinal curves and health. *J Manipulative Physiol Ther.* 2008 Nov-Dec; 31(9): 690–714.

14   Panjabi (1992) The Stabilizing System of the Spine. Part I. Function, Dysfunction, Adaptation, and Enhancement. *Journal of Spinal Disorders and Techniques.* Vol. 5, No. 4 1992; http://appliedspine.redhawk-tech.com/ Medical-Professionals-and-Physicians/White-Papers/The_stabilizing_ system_of_the_spine_part_1.pdf

15   Schmidt, Lee (2005) *Motor Control and Learning: A Behavioral Emphasis.* p. 53.

16   Schachter (2011). *Psychology.*

17   Proske and Gandevia (2012) The Proprioceptive Senses: Their Roles in Signaling Body Shape, Body Position and Movement, and Muscle Force. *Physiol Rev.* October 1, 2012, 92 (4), 1651–1697. http://physrev.physiology.org/ content/92/4/1651.full.pdf+html

[18] Shumway-Cook, Woollcott (2012) p. 4.

[19] Shumway-Cook, Woolacott (2012) p. 16.

[20] Shumway-Cook, Woolacott (2012) p. 51

[21] Shumway-Cook, Woolacott (2012) p. 27.

[22] Shumway-Cook, Woolacott (2012) p. 27.

[23] Schmidt, Lee (2005) p. 162.

[24] Shumway-Cook, Woolacott (2012) p. 51, 17.

[25] I will often refer to this brain activity as "neural" activity, but in fact the function of the brain depends on other structures, including glial cells.

[26] For an accessible review see Doidge (2008) *The Brain that Changes Itself,* or Blaskeslee (2008) *The Body has a Mind of its Own.*

[27] Ramachandran and Ramachandran (2000) Phantom Limbs and Neural Plasticity, *Arch Neurol.* 2000; 57 (3): 317–320.

[28] Pascual-Leone (2001) The brain that plays music and is changed by it. *Ann N Y Acad Sci.* 2001 Jun; 930: 315–29.

[29] Pascual-Leone A, Torres F. (1998) Plasticity of the sensorimotor cortex representation of the reading finger in Braille readers. *Brain.* 1993; 116 (1): 39–52; Hamilton, Pascual-Leone (1998) Cortical plasticity associated with Braille learning. *Trends in Cognitive Sciences,* Vol. 2, Issue 5, 1 May 1998, 168–174.

[30] Id.

[31] Quote from interview on youtube: https://www.youtube.com/watch?v=rupZ-wlRdA0

[32] Kerr and Shaw (2008) Tactile acuity in experienced Tai Chi practitioners: evidence for use dependent plasticity as an effect of sensory-attentional training. *Experimental Brain Research.* June 2008, Vol. 188, Issue 2, 317–322. http://www.ncbi.nlm.nih.gov/pmc/articles/PMC2795804

[33] Allard, Clark, Jenkins, Merzenich (1991) Reorganization of somatosensory area 3b representations in adult owl monkeys after digital syndactyly. AJP — *JN Physiol.* September 1, 1991, vol. 66, no. 3, 1048–1058. http://jn.physiology.org/content/66/3/1048.abstract

34   When a part of the brain goes unused (as would be the case with the part of the brain controlling a phantom limb), other parts will start to cannibalize it like dandelions moving into a field.

35   Pascual-Leone, Amir Amedi (2005) The Plastic Human Brain Cortex, *Annu. Rev. Neurosci.* 2005. 28: 377–401. http://www.annualreviews.org/doi/pdf/10.1146/annurev.neuro.27.070203.144216

36   Id.

37   Picard, Matsuzaka, Strick (2013) Extended practice of a motor skill is associated with reduced metabolic activity in M1. *Nature Neuroscience* 16, 1340–1347.

38   Wiestler, Diedrichsen (2013) Skill learning strengthens cortical representations of motor sequences. *Elife*. 2013 Jul 9. http://www.ncbi.nlm.nih.gov/pmc/articles/PMC3707182/pdf/elife00801.pdf

39   Shumway-Cook, Woolacott (2012), p. 92.

40   Chabrirs and Simons (2011) *The Invisible Gorilla: How Our Intuitions Deceive Us*

41   Attention seems to work at the level of the synapse, strengthening certain connections and inhibiting others. Farran Briggs, George R. Mangun, W. Martin Usrey (2013) Attention enhances synaptic efficacy and the signal-to-noise ratio in neural circuits. *Nature*, 2013; 499 (7459).

42   Attention amplifies neural activity associated with the sensory input to which attention is directed. Kerr and Shaw (2008) Tactile acuity in experienced Tai Chi practitioners: evidence for use dependent plasticity as an effect of sensory-attentional training. *Experimental Brain Research*, June 2008, Vol. 188, Issue 2, 317–322. http://www.ncbi.nlm.nih.gov/pmc/articles/PMC2795804

43   Focus increases the efficacy of perceptual training. Seitz & Dinse, 2007. A common framework for perceptual learning. *Curr Opin Neurobiol*. 2007 Apr; 17(2): 148–53. Epub 2007 Feb 20.

44   Wulf (2007) *Attention and Motor Skill Learning.*

[45] Schmidt, Lee (2005) p. 115.

[46] Downar, Crawley, et al. (2000) A multimodal cortical network for the detection of changes in the sensory environment. *Nature Neuroscience.* 3, (2000) 277–283.

[47] Paul Ingraham (2009) Does Ultrasound Work? http://saveyourself.ca/articles/ultrasound.php

[48] Bystrom, et al. (2013) Motor Control Exercises Reduces Pain and Disability in Chronic and Recurrent Low Back Pain: A Meta-Analysis. *Spine:* 15 March 2013, Vol. 38, Issue 6, E350–E358.

[49] Moseley, Flor (2012) Targeting Cortical Representations in the Treatment of Pain. *Neurorehabil Neural Repair.* 2012 Jul–Aug; 26(6): 646–52.

[50] Shumway-Cook, Woolacott (2012) p. 28.

[51] Wolpert, Flanagan (2001) Motor Prediction. http://wexler.free.fr/library/files/wolpert%20%282001%29%20motor%20prediction.pdf

[52] Ratey, Hagerman (2008) *Spark: The Revolutionary New Science of Exercise and the Brain.*

[53] Shumway-Cook, Woolacott (2012) pp. 195–197.

[54] Some of these patterns are more fundamental than others. Although some children learn to walk without ever having crawled, none will learn either without learning to stabilize the head.

[55] Flash and Hochner (2005) Motor Primitives in Vertebrates and Invertebrates. Current opinion in *Neurobiology* 15 (6): 660–666. http://e.guigon.free.fr/rsc/article/FlashHochner05.pdf

[56] Id.

[57] Shumway-Cook, Woolacott (2012) p. 32.

[58] Garvey, C. (1990). *Play.* Cambridge, MA: Harvard University Press.

[59] Gordon, Burke (2003) Socially-induced brain "fertilization": play promotes brain derived neurotrophic factor transcription in the amygdala and dorsolateral frontal cortex in juvenile rats. *Neurosci Lett.* 2003 Apr 24; 341(1): 17–20. http://www.ncbi.nlm.nih.gov/pubmed/12676333

[60] Fares, et al. (2013) Standardized environmental enrichment supports enhanced brain plasticity in healthy rats and prevents cognitive impairment in epileptic rats. *PLoS One.* 2013; 8(1): e53888. http://www.ncbi.nlm.nih.gov/pubmed/23342033

[61] Taking Play Seriously, *The New York Times.* http://www.nytimes.com/2008/02/17/magazine/17play.html?pagewanted=all&_r=0

[62] Id.

[63] Dr. Michael Merzenich on Neuroscience, Learning and the Feldenkrais Method(R), youtube video. http://www.youtube.com/watch?v=rupZ-wlRdA0

[64] Moseley, Butler (2013) *Explain Pain;* Melzack, Wall (2004) *The Challenge of Pain.*

[65] Mosely (2003) A Pain Neuromatrix Approach to Patients in Chronic Pain. *Man Ther.* 2003 Aug; 8(3): 130-40. http://www.ncbi.nlm.nih.gov/pubmed/12909433

[66] Id.

[67] Dimsdale, Dantzer (2007) A biological substrate for somatoform disorders. *Psychosom Med* 2007 Dec. 69(9): 850-854 http://www.ncbi.nlm.nih.gov/pmc/articles/PMC2908292/

[68] Geuter, et al. (2013) Facilitation of Pain in the Human Spinal Cord by Nocebo Treatment. *The Journal of Neuroscience.* 21 August 2013; 33(34): 13784-13790. http://www.jneurosci.org/content/33/34/13784

[69] Smith et al. (1998) The meaning of pain: cancer patients rating and recall of pain intensity and affect. *Pain.* 1998; 78: 123-9.

[70] Moseley (2003) Joining forces — combining cognition-targeted motor control training with group or individual pain physiology education: a successful treatment for chronic low back pain. *J Manip Therap.* 2003; 11:88-94.

[71] Moseley (2011) TEDX Adelaide: *Why Things Hurt.* http://www.youtube.com/watch?v=gwd-wLdIHjs

[72] Lumley, Cohen et al. (2011) Pain and emotion: a biopsychosocial review of recent research. *J Clin Psychol.* 2011; 67:1–27

[73] Mosely (2013) *Explain Pain.* p. 21.

[74] Jensen et al. (1994) MRI of the lumbar spine in people without back pain. *N Engl J Med.* 1994 Jul 14; 331(2): 69–73. http://www.ncbi.nlm.nih.gov/pubmed/8208267

[75] Boden et al. (1990) Abnormal magnetic-resonance scans of the lumbar spine in asymptomatic subjects. A prospective investigation. *J Bone Joint Surg Am.* 1990 Mar; 72(3): 403–8. http://www.ncbi.nlm.nih.gov/pubmed/2312537.

[76] American Orthopaedic Society for Sports Medicine (2010). http://phys.org/news187851086.html

[77] Beattie et al. (2005) Abnormalities identified in the knees of asymptomatic volunteers using peripheral magnetic resonance imaging. *Osteoarthritis Cartilage.* 2005 Mar; 13(3): 181–6. http://www.ncbi.nlm.nih.gov/pubmed/15727883

[78] Templehof et al. (1999) Age-related prevalence of rotator cuff tears in asymptomatic shoulders. *Journal of Shoulder and Elbow Surgery* Vol. 8, Issue 4, July 1999, 296–299. http://www.jshoulderelbow.org/article/S1058-2746%2899%2990148-9/abstract

[79] Connor, Banks et al. (2003) Magnetic Resonance Imaging of the Asymptomatic Shoulder of Overhead Athletes. A 5-Year Follow-up Study. *Am J Sports Med* September 2003, Vol. 31, No. 5, 724–727. http://ajs.sagepub.com/content/31/5/724.short

[80] Moseley (2007) Painful Yarns: Metaphors & Stories to Help Understand the Biology of Pain. p. 34.

[81] Moseley (2008) Reconceptualising Placebo. *BMJ.* 2008 May 17; 336(7653): 1086. http://www.ncbi.nlm.nih.gov/pmc/articles/PMC2386632/

[82] Humphrey and Skoles (2012) The evolutionary psychology of healing: A human success story. *Current Biology.* Vol. 22, Issue 17, 11 September 2012, R695–R698. http://www.sciencedirect.com/science/article/pii/S096098221200663X

[83] Moseley (2013) *Explain Pain,* p. 30

[84] Id., p. 36.

[85] Id.

[86] Id.

[87] Id.; Woolf (2000) Central Sensitization: Implications for the Diagnosis and Treatment of pain. *Pain.* 2011 March; 152 (3 Suppl): S2–15. http://www.ncbi

.nlm.nih.gov/pmc/articles/PMC3268359/; Van Wilgen et al. (2012) The sensitization model to explain how chronic pain exists without tissue damage. *Pain Manag Nurs.* 2012 Mar; 13(1): 60–5. http://www.painmanagementnursing. org/article/S1524-9042%2810%2900032-9/fulltext

[88] Id.

[89] Id.

[90] Id.

[91] Bove et al. (2003) Inflammation induces ectopic mechanical sensitivity in axons of nociceptors innervating deep tissues. *J Neurophysiol.* 2003 Sep; 90(3): 1949–55. http://www.ncbi.nlm.nih.gov/pubmed/12724363.

[92] Id.; Butler (2006) *Sensitive Nervous System.*

[93] Butler (2006) *Sensitive Nervous System,* p. 81.

[94] Geuter, et al. (2013) Facilitation of Pain in the Human Spinal Cord by Nocebo Treatment. *The Journal of Neuroscience.* 21 August 2013, 33(34): 13784–13790. http://www.jneurosci.org/content/33/34/13784

[95] Butler (2013) Youtube video. The Drug Cabinet in the Brain. http://www .youtube.com/watch?v=Gd2NaGZa7M4

[96] Yarnitsky (2010) Conditioned pain modulation (the diffuse noxious inhibitory control-like effect): its relevance for acute and chronic pain states. Current Opinion in *Anaesthesiology.* October 2010, Vol. 23, Issue 5; 611–615. http://journals.lww.com/coanesthesiology/Abstract/2010/10000/ Conditioned_pain_modulation__the_diffuse_noxious.14.aspx

[97] Goffaux et al. (2007) Descending analgesia: When the spine echoes what the brain expects. *Pain.* Vol. 130, Issues 1–2, July 2007; 137–143. http://www .sciencedirect.com/science/article/pii/S0304395906006439.

[98] Melzack and Katz (2012) Pain. Wiley Interdisciplinary Reviews: *Cognitive Science.* January/February 2013, Vol. 4, Issue 1; 1–15. http://online library.wiley.com/doi/10.1002/wcs.1201/full

[99] Moseley and Butler (2013) *Explain Pain* pp. 38; 76–78.

[100] Moseley Flor (2012) Targeting cortical representations in the treatment of chronic pain: a review. *Neurorehabil Neural Repair.* 2012 Jul–Aug; 26(6): 646–52. http://www.bodyinmind.org/wp-content/uploads/Moseley-Flor-2012-Neurorehab-Neural-Rep-targeting-the-brain-in-rehab-review.pdf

[101] Id.

[102] Moseley, Butler, Beames (2012) *The Graded Motor Imagery Handbook.*

[103] Moseley, Flor (2012) Targeting cortical representations in the treatment of chronic pain: a review. *Neurorehabil Neural Repair.* 2012 Jul-Aug; 26(6): 646–52. http://www.bodyinmind.org/wp-content/uploads/Moseley-Flor-2012-Neurorehab-Neural-Rep-targeting-the-brain-in-rehab-review.pdf

[104] Id.

[105] Id; Lotze Moseley (2007) Role of Distorted Body Image in Pain. *Current Rheumatology Reports* 2007, Sept; 9:488–496. http://www.bodyinmind.org/wp-content/uploads/Lotze-Moseley-2007-Curr-Rheum-Reports-distorted-image-and-pain1.pdf

[106] Barnsley et al. (2011) *Current Biology.* Vol. 21, Issue 23, 6 December 2011; R945–R946. http://www.sciencedirect.com/science/article/pii/S0960982211012000

[107] Id.

[108] Moseley (2008) I can't find it! Distorted body image and tactile dysfunction in patients with chronic back pain. *Pain.* (2008) 140, 239–243. http://www.bodyinmind.org/wp-content/uploads/Moseley-2008-PAIN-i-cant-find-it.pdf

[109] Moseley (2012) Spatially defined modulation of skin temperature and hand ownership of both hands in patients with unilateral complex regional pain syndrome. *Brain.* 2012 Dec; 135(Pt 12): 3676–86. http://www.ncbi.nlm.nih.gov/pubmed/23250885

[110] Moseley, Galagher et al. (2012) Neglect-like tactile dysfunction in chronic back pain. *Neurology.* 2012 Jul 24; 79(4): 327–32. http://www.ncbi.nlm.nih.gov/pubmed/22744662

[111] McCabe, Cohen et al. (2007) Somaesthetic disturbances in fibromyalgia are exaggerated by sensory–motor conflict: implications for chronicity of the disease? *Rheumatology* (2007) 46 (10): 1587–1592. http://rheumatology.oxfordjournals.org/content/46/10/1587.full. But note that other studies have been

unable to increase pain in healthy volunteers with sensory motor mismatch. For example: Wand, et. al. (2014) Moving in an Environment at Induced Sensorimotor Incongruence Does not Influence Pain Sensitivity in Health Volunteers. PLoS ONE 9(4): e93701.

[112] Kammers et al. (2010) Cooling the thermal-grill illusion through self-touch. *Curr Biol.* 2010 Oct 26; 20(20): 1819–22. http://www.ncbi.nlm.nih.gov/pubmed/20869246

[113] Wand, et al. (2012) Seeing It Helps. movement-related back pain is reduced by visualization of the back during movement. *Clin J Pain.* 2012 Sep; 28(7): 602–8. http://www.ncbi.nlm.nih.gov/pubmed/22699134

[114] Moseley and Butler (2013) *Explain Pain.*

[115] Lederman (2010) The fall of the postural–structural–biomechanical model in manual and physical therapies: Exemplified by lower back pain CPDO *Online Journal* (2010), March, p. 1–14.

[116] Luouw et al. (2011) The effect of neuroscience education on pain, disability, anxiety, and stress in chronic musculoskeletal pain. *Archives of Physical Medicine and Rehabilitation.* December 2011, Vol. 92, Issue 12, 2041–2056. http://www.archives-pmr.org/article/S0003-9993(11)00670-8/fulltext

[117] Moseley, Flor (2012) Targeting cortical representations in the treatment of chronic pain: a review. *Neurorehabil Neural Repair.* 2012 Jul-Aug; 26(6): 646–52. http://www.bodyinmind.org/wp-content/uploads/Moseley-Flor-2012-Neurorehab-Neural-Rep-targeting-the-brain-in-rehab-review.pdf; Budreau et al. (2010) The role of motor learning and neuroplasticity in designing rehabilitation approaches for musculoskeletal pain disorders. *Manual Therapy.* 15 (2010) 410–414. http://ispje.org/showcase2010/Manual%20Therapy%20Showcase%20article2010.pdf

[118] Bystrom et al. (2013) Motor control exercises reduces pain and disability in chronic and recurrent low back pain: a meta-analysis. *Spine.* 15 March 2013; Vol. 38, Issue 6, E350–E358. http://journals.lww.com/spinejournal/Abstract/2013/03150/Motor_Control_Exercises_Reduces_Pain_and.18.aspx

[119] http://en.wikipedia.org/wiki/Sensory_gating

[120] Article in *Scientific American*. http://www.scientificamerican.com/article .cfm?id=extreme-fear-superhuman&page=2

[121] Hasaan et al. (2002) Effect of pain reduction on postural sway, proprioception, and quadriceps strength in subjects with knee osteoarthritis. *Ann Rheum Dis* 2002; 61: 422–428. http://ard.bmj.com/content/61/5/422. abstract; Henriksen (2007) Experimental knee pain reduces muscle strength. *The Journal of Pain*. April 2011, Vol. 12, Issue 4, 460–467, http://www .jpain.org/article/S1526-5900(10)00760-1/abstract

[122] Makofsky (2007) Immediate effect of grade iv inferior hip joint mobilization on hip abductor torque: a pilot study. *J Man Manip Ther.* 2007; 15(2): 103–110. http://www.ncbi.nlm.nih.gov/pmc/articles/PMC2565609/

[123] Weppler et al. (2010) Increasing muscle extensibility: a matter of increasing length or modifying sensation? *Phys Ther.* 2010 Mar; 90(3): 438–49. http://www .ncbi.nlm.nih.gov/pubmed/20075147; Ben, Harvey (2010) Regular stretch does not increase muscle extensibility: a randomized controlled trial. *Scandinavian Journal of Medicine and Science in Sports*. Feb 2010; 20(1): 136–144.

[124] Noakes (2012) Fatigue is a brain-derived emotion that regulates the exercise behavior to ensure the protection of whole body homeostasis. *Front Physiol*. 2012; 3: 82. http://www.ncbi.nlm.nih.gov/pmc/articles/PMC3323922/?tool=pubmed.

[125] Id.

[126] Id.

[127] Hodges (2011) Pain and motor control: From the laboratory to rehabilitation. *Journal of Electromyography and Kinesiology* 21 (2011) 220–228. http://fbeosteo .com/wp-content/uploads/Painandmotor.pdf;

[128] Id.

[129] Hodges (2011) Moving differently in pain: a new theory to explain the adaptation to pain. *Pain*. 2011 Mar; 152(3 Suppl): S90–8. http://fbeosteo.com/ wp-content/uploads/Painandmotor.pdf

[130] Carney (2010) Power posing: brief nonverbal displays affect neuroendocrine levels and risk tolerance. *Psychol Sci*. 2010 Oct; 21(10): 1363–8. http://www.ncbi .nlm.nih.gov/pubmed/20855902.

Huang, et al. (2011) Powerful postures versus powerful roles. which is the proximate correlate of thought and behavior? *Psychological Science.* Jan 2011, Vol. 22, No. 1, 95–102. http://pss.sagepub.com/content/22/1/95

[131] Strack (1988) Inhibiting and facilitating conditions of the human smile: a nonobtrusive test of the facial feedback hypothesis. *J Pers Soc Psychol.* 1988 May; 54(5): 768–77.

[132] Davis et al. (2010) The effects of botox injections on emotional experience. *Emotion.* 2010 June 10(3): 433–440. http://www.ncbi.nlm.nih.gov/pmc/articles/PMC2880828/

[133] Cook et al. (2007) Making children gesture brings out implicit knowledge and leads to learning. *J Exp Psychol Gen.* 2007 Nov; 136(4): 539–50. http://www.ncbi.nlm.nih.gov/pubmed/17999569

[134] Cheg Bo-Zhong et al. (2006) Washing away your sins: threatened morality and physical cleansing. *Science.* 8 September 2006: Vol. 313, No. 5792, 1451–1452. http://www.sciencemag.org/content/313/5792/1451.abstract

[135] Casasanto D, Jasmin K (2010) Good and bad in the hands of politicians: spontaneous gestures during positive and negative speech. PLoS ONE 5(7): e11805. doi:10.1371/journal.pone.0011805

[136] Speirer et al. (2013) Training-induced behavioral and brain plasticity in inhibitory control. *Frontiers in Human Neuroscience.* Aug 2013; 7, Article 427.

[137] Verbruggen et al. (2012) Proactive motor control reduces monetary risk taken in gambling. *Psychological Science.* 23(7): 805–815. http://psych.cf.ac.uk/home2/chambers/Verbruggen_2012_PsychScience.pdf.

[138] Id.

[139] Id.

[140] Kerr, Sachett, et al. (2013) Mindfulness starts with the body: somatosensory attention and top-down modulation of cortical alpha rhythms in mindfulness meditation. *Frontiers of Human Neuroscience.* Feb 13, 2013.

[141] Zeidan, Martucci, et al. Brain mechanisms supporting the modulation of pain by mindfulness meditation. *The Journal of Neuroscience.* Apr 6, 2011; 31(14): 5540–5548. http://www.jneurosci.org/content/31/14/5540.full.pdf+html

[142] Emerson, Zeidan (et al. (2013) Pain sensitivity is inversely related to regional grey matter density in the brain. *J. Pain.* 2013 12 004. http://www .painjournalonline.com/article/S0304-3959(13)00641-6/abstract; http://www .sciencedaily.com/releases/2014/01/140114114136.htm

[143] Id.

[144] Id.

[145] Craig (2003) Interoception: the sense of the physiological condition of the body. Current Opinion in *Neurobiology.* 2003, 13: 500–505. http://www.jsmf .org/meetings/2007/oct-nov/CONB%20Craig%202003.pdf

[146] Pollatos, Kirsch, et al. (2005) On the relationship between interoceptive awareness, emotional experience, and brain processes. *Cognitive Brain Research* 25 (2005) 948–962. http://www.i3.psychologie.uni-wuerzburg .de/fileadmin/06020300/user_upload/pollatos__kirsch__schandry__ CognBrainRes__2005.pdf.

[147] Id.

[148] Researchers Study Self-Knowledge (Literally) The Body Sends Cues to the Brain; Understanding Them Can Improve Your Health, *Wall Street Journal,* August 26, 2013. http://online.wsj.com/news/articles/SB10001424127887324 5912045790367521200097292?mg=reno64-wsj&url=http%3A%2F%2Fonline.wsj .com%2Farticle%2FSB1000142412788732459120457903675212009729.html

[149] Id.

[150] Id.

CPSIA information can be obtained at www.ICGtesting.com
Printed in the USA
LVOW05s2254220315

431598LV00007B/55/P